Health Services in
the United States

Health Services in the United States

Florence A. Wilson   Duncan Neuhauser

Ballinger Publishing Company • Cambridge, Mass.
A Subsidiary of J.B. Lippincott Company

International Standard Book Number: 0-88410-101-0

Library of Congress Catalog Card Number: 73-22396

Printed in the United States of America

Library of Congress Cataloging in Publication Data

Wilson, Florence A
      Health services in the United States.

      1. Medical care—United States. I. Neuhauser, Duncan, joint author.
II. Title. [DNLM: 1. Delivery of health care—U.S. WB50 AA1W7h 1974]
RA395.A3W54   362.1'0973   73-22396
ISBN 0-88410-101-0

Table of Contents

List of Figures   ix

List of Tables   xi

Preface   xiii

Chapter One
Health Care Institutions   1

1. Introduction   1
2. Hospitals (1)   5
3. Hospitals (2)   13
4. Hospital Departments and Services   17
5. Joint Commission on Accreditation of Hospitals (JCAH)   25
6. Nursing Homes   29
7. Other Health Services   31
8. Regulation of Health Services Institutions   34

Chapter Two
Health Manpower   41

1. Overview   41
2. Physicians   58
3. Dentists   65
4. Nurses   66
5. A Sampling of Other Health Professions   70

Chapter Three
Paying for Care   77

1. Introduction   77
2. Health Insurance and Prepayment   80

3. Health Plans, HMOs   87
4. Financing   89

Chapter Four
The Federal Government and Health Care   101

1. The Federal Government and Health: Overview   101
2. The Department of Health, Education and Welfare   104
3. Introduction to Health Legislation   117
4. The Social Security Act   121
5. Social Security Amendments of 1960–"Kerr-Mills Act"   124
6. Maternal and Child Health and Mental Retardation
        Planning Amendments of 1963   125
7. Social Security Amendments of 1965–"Medicare," "Medicaid"   126
8. Medicare and Medicaid Amendments of 1966-1971   136
9. Social Security Amendments of 1972–"HR-1"   138
10. Summary of Medicare   143
11. Summary of Medicaid   145
12. Summary of Social Security Act Titles   146
13. The Public Health Service Act   147
14. Hospital Survey and Construction Act of 1946–"Hill-Burton Act"   152
15. Heart Disease, Cancer and Stroke Amendments of 1965–"Regional
        Medical Programs"   155
16. Comprehensive Health Planning and Public Health Service
        Amendments of 1966–"Partnership for Health"   158
17. Health Manpower Legislation Under the Public Health
        Service Act   161
18. Health Maintenance Organization Act of 1973   166
19. Summary of Public Health Service Act Titles   169
20. Mental Retardation Facilities and Community Mental Health
        Centers Construction Act of 1963   171
21. Summary of Mental Retardation and Mental Health Center
        Titles   174
22. Economic Opportunity Act of 1964–"Anti-Poverty Program"   175
    A Note to the Reader   177

Chapter Five
State and Local Health Activities   179

Chapter Six
Ambulatory Care (Non-Institutional Care)   183

Chapter Seven
Voluntary Agencies   191

Chapter Eight
Review and Control of Quality and Costs 193

1. Quality Control 193
2. Cost Control 195

Chapter Nine
The Pharmaceutical Industry 199

1. Drugs 199
2. The Structure of the Prescription Industry 201

Appendixes

Appendix A Alphabet Soup 205
Appendix B Chronological List of Laws 209

Index 213

List of Figures

1-1. Types of Hospital Ownership 5

3-1. Payment for Health Services—Schematic Diagram of Flow of
Funds (Simplified) 91

3-2. National Health Expenditures and Percentage of Gross National
Product, Selected Fiscal Years, 1950–72 92

3-3. Distribution of Personal Health Care Expenditures, by Source
of Funds and Type of Expenditure, Fiscal Year 1972 100

List of Tables

1-1. An Example of an Organization Chart for a Large Community General Hospital ... 18

1-2. The Progress of a Herniorrhaphy Patient Through a Community General Hospital
       Part I ... 26
       Part II ... 27
       Part III ... 28

1-3. Nursing and Related Homes Recognized Under Government Programs ... 29

1-4. Revised Classification of Nursing Homes Recognized Under Government Programs Since June 1973 ... 30

1-5. Hospitals and Hospital Beds: Selected Years 1963 through 1970 ... 32

1-6. Ownership of Hospitals: 1970 ... 33

1-7. Ownership of Nursing Care and Related Homes: 1969 ... 33

1-8. Inpatient Health Facilities: Selected Years 1963 through 1970 ... 34

1-9. Beds in Inpatient Health Facilities: Selected Years 1963 through 1970 ... 35

1-10. Typology of Regulation ... 36

2-1. List of Health Occupations ... 43

2-2. Estimated Persons Employed in Selected Occupations Within Each Health Field: 1970 ... 50

2-3. Accrediting Agencies for Educational Programs ... 54

2-4. Calendar for Health Career Education ... 56

2-5. Modal Physician's Progress ... 60

2-6. Type of Practice and Primary Specialty of Active Federal and Non-Federal Physicians: 1967 and 1970 ... 63

3-1.   Aggregate and Per Capita National Health Expenditures,
        by Source of Funds and Percentage of Gross National Product
        Selected Fiscal Years, 1928-29 through 1971-72   93

3-2.   National Health Expenditures, by Type of Expenditure and
        Source of Funds, Fiscal Years 1969-70 through 1971-72   94

3-3.   Expenditures for Health Services and Supplies under
        Public Programs, by Program, Type of Expenditures, and
        Source of Funds, Fiscal Year 1971-72   96

3-4.   Aggregate and Per Capita National Health Expenditures,
        by Type of Expenditure, Selected Fiscal Years, 1928-29
        through 1971-72   98

4-1.   Department of Health, Education and Welfare, 1953   105

4-2.   Department of Health, Education and Welfare, 1972   110

4-3.   Health Services and Mental Health Administration, 1972   111

4-4.   Department of Health, Education, and Welfare, 1974   112

Preface

This description of health services in the United States was originally developed for graduate students at the Harvard School of Public Health. It attempts to provide a concise summary of major components of health care in this country. Much of this information has only been available in widely scattered, often elusive documents, or exists as common knowledge among health professionals who learned it by experience or word of mouth.

One might refer to this document as the anatomy of American health services. It stops short of being physiology, that is, how the system works. It stops short of being pathology, that is, how and where the services fail to work. Finally, it does not include the techniques which managers, professionals, or consumers might use to operate, modify or change health services.

We have attempted to be as objective and dispassionate as possible. However, this is often exceedingly difficult. One can scarcely write a word in this field without it being the potential source of controversy and debate. For example, take the title of this document. We might have referred to the "U.S. Health Services System," but there is an argument as to whether it is a "system" or a "non-system." The social scientists refer to it as a "system," implying that it has a boundary, component parts, and relationships. The reformers refer to it as a "non-system" implying that it is chaotic and in need of a reorganization along more rational lines.* We have tried to avoid taking sides but since much of the content has been the focus of political or ideological debates the task is difficult.

A document such as this has other inherent problems. For example, much effort has gone into making it as brief as possible, which leads to the dilemma of what to include and what to exclude and where to place the emphasis.

---

*We might have used health services industry instead of system, but one ideological implication of the word "industry" is that health services are just like the automobile or steel industry and they are or should be all under the control of the market place.

Here our general rule has been to focus on those areas which are most important to the understanding of current issues. Some readers therefore may feel that their own occupation or organization has not been covered to the depth they would like. Also, since one of the distinguishing characteristics of American health services is their great diversity and variety, many general descriptive statements may be to some degree misleading or wrong; yet, if every exception were cited this document would be unduly long. Finally, some of the material will soon be affected by ongoing changes in laws and institutions. Despite these problems, we hope this endeavor will prove useful.

Comments, criticisms and suggestions concerning this initial endeavor will be welcomed, and may be communicated directly to the authors. The first two chapters, most of the third, and the eighth were done by D.N. The remaining chapters, and section on nurses, are by F.W.

Finally, we wish to express our appreciation to the Ford Foundation Urban Studies Seminar for assistance in the development of this book.

Harvard School of Public Health   Duncan Neuhauser, Ph.D.
Boston   Florence A. Wilson, M.D.

Chapter One

Health Care Institutions

1. INTRODUCTION

Types of Health Care Institutions
(Organizations, Facilities)

There is a wide variety of health facilities which vary according to type of patient served and the extent of services provided.

Inpatient and Residential
A. Inpatient Care (having permanent facilities, beds, medical services and continuous nursing services)
   1. Hospitals, general and special, short and long stay (having a medical staff and organized physician services)
   2. Nursing Homes
      Extended Care Institution, Extended Care Facility (ECF)
      Skilled Nursing Care Institution
      Intermediate Care Institution
B. Health-Related Care Institutions (for patients whose primary needs are personal care, sheltered care, or adaptive services)
   1. Personal Care Institutions (providing personal services related to activities of daily living)
   2. Sheltered Care Institutions (providing protective environment and occasional personal care services)
C. Domiciliary Institutions (living accommodations without health-related services)
   Special housing for the aged
D. Other Specialized Facilities
   Facilities for the deaf and blind (homes and schools)
   Facilities for unwed mothers
   Facilities for the mentally retarded

Facilities for dependent children and orphans
Facilities for drug addicts
Homes for alcoholics
Juvenile correctional facilities

Nonpatient Facilities (providing goods and services, but not directly to patients)
A.   Clinical (medical) laboratories
Dental laboratories
Optician establishments
B.   Pharmaceutical manufacturers and distributors
C.   Hospital supply industry
D.   Insurance companies, Blue Cross and Blue Shield

The following three definitions are used by the American Hospital Association.[1] Other definitions exist. Drawing the line between different types of facilities is somewhat arbitrary because the boundary lines are not completely clear.

General Hospitals

Definition.   Establishments with organized medical staffs; with permanent facilities that include inpatient beds; and with medical services, including physician services and continuous nursing services, to provide diagnosis and treatment for patients who have a variety of medical conditions, both surgical and nonsurgical.

Essential Characteristics for Classification
1.   The primary function of the institution is to provide diagnostic and treatment services for patients who have a variety of medical conditions, both surgical and nonsurgical.
2.   The institution maintains inpatient beds.
3.   There is a governing authority legally responsible for the conduct of the institution.
4.   There is an administrator to whom the governing authority delegates the full-time responsibility for the operation of the institution in accordance with established policy.
5.   There is an organized medical staff to which the governing authority delegates responsibility for maintaining proper standards of medical care.
6.   Each patient is admitted on the medical authority of, and is under the supervision of, a member of the medical staff.

---

[1] American Hospital Association, *Classification of Health Care Institutions,* Chicago, 1968 edition.

7. Registered professional nurse supervision and other nursing services are continuous.
8. A current and complete medical record is maintained for each patient.
9. Pharmacy service is maintained in the institution and is supervised by a registered pharmacist.
10. Diagnostic X-ray service, with facilities and staff for a variety of procedures, is maintained in the institution.
11. Clinical laboratory service, with facilities and staff for a variety of tests and procedures, is maintained in the institution, and anatomical pathology services are regularly and conveniently available.
12. Operating room service, with facilities and staff, is maintained in the institution.
13. Food served to patients meets their nutritional requirements, and special diets are regularly available.

General Extended Care Institutions[2]

Definition. Establishments with organized medical staffs; with permanent facilities that include inpatient beds; and with medical services, including physician services and continuous nursing services, to provide treatment for patients who require inpatient care but are not in an acute phase of illness, who currently require primarily convalescent or restorative services, and who have a variety of medical conditions.

Essential Characteristics for Classification
1. The primary function of the institution is to provide treatment for patients who require inpatient care, but who are not in an acute phase of illness, who currently require primarily convalescent or restorative services, and who have a variety of medical conditions.
2. There are arrangements for transfer of patients in need of hospital care.
3. The institution maintains inpatient beds.
4. There is a governing authority legally responsible for the conduct of the institution.
5. There is an administrator to whom the governing authority delegates the full-time responsibility for the operation of the institution in accordance with established policy.
6. One or more physicians are responsible for advising the governing authority on proper standards of medical care.

---

[2] See section on *Nursing Homes.*

7. Each patient is admitted on the medical authority of, and is under the supervision of, a physician.
8. A current and complete medical record is maintained for each patient.
9. Registered professional nurse supervision and other nursing services are continuous.
10. Diagnostic X-ray service and clinical laboratory service are regularly and conveniently available.
11. There is control of the storage and dispensing of narcotics and other medications.
12. Food served to patients meets their nutritional requirements, and special diets are regularly available.

General Nursing Care Institutions

Definition. Establishments with *permanent facilities* that include inpatient beds; and with medical services, including continuous nursing services, to provide treatment for patients who require inpatient care but do not currently require continuous hospital services, and who have a variety of medical conditions.

Essential Characteristics for Classification
1. The primary function of the institution is to provide treatment services for patients who require inpatient care but do not currently require continuous hospital services, and who have a variety of medical conditions.
2. There are arrangements for transfer of patients in need of hospital care.
3. The institution maintains inpatient beds.
4. There is a governing authority legally responsible for the conduct of the institution.
5. There is an administrator to whom the governing authority delegates the full-time responsibility for the operation of the institution in accordance with established policy.
6. One or more physicians is responsible for advising the governing authority on proper standards of medical care.
7. Each patient is admitted on the medical authority of, and is under the supervision of, a physician.
8. A current and complete medical record is maintained for each patient.
9. The nursing services are under the supervision of a full-time registered professional nurse; licensed graduate nurse supervision and other nursing services are continuous.
10. There are arrangements for obtaining necessary clinical laboratory and diagnostic X-ray services.

11. There is control of the storage and dispensing of narcotics and other medications.
12. Food served to patients meets their nutritional requirements, and special diets are regularly available.

2. HOSPITALS (1)

Hospitals can be characterized in a number of different ways, including:

1. Ownership
2. Type of Patient Treated and Services Provided
3. Average Length of Patient Stay
4. Medical and Osteopathic
5. Teaching and Non-Teaching.

The American hospital system provides an incredibly wide variety of types of hospitals; the most important in terms of volume of patients cared for are the state long-term mental hospitals and the voluntary short-term general community hospitals.

Because there are so many variations according to types of ownership, organization, and types of patient treated, there are numerous exceptions to what follows.

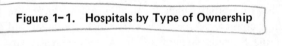

Figure 1-1. Hospitals by Type of Ownership

Government Ownership

Private (Non-Government) Ownership

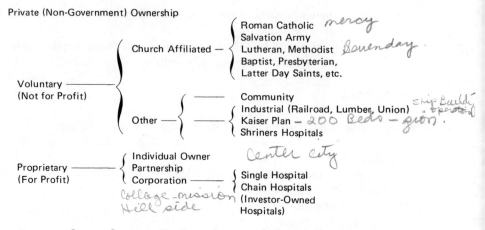

Source: James A. Hamilton, *Patterns of Hospital Ownership and Control*, (Minneapolis: University of Minnesota Press, 1961).

Hospital Ownership

Federal

Army.   These hospitals are administratively separated into (a) overseas hospitals, and (b) continental U.S. (CONUS) hospitals; the CONUS hospitals are divided into Class I hospitals which are smaller and are under the command of the regional army commander, and Class II, which are larger and are under the jurisdiction of the Surgeon General of the Army. Their primary role is to care for army personnel and secondarily to provide care for army personnel dependents (wives and children).

Navy.   For navy and marine corps personnel and dependents.

Air Force.   For air force personnel and dependents.

Veteran's Administration.   Provides the largest unified health service system in the U.S., consisting of 167 hospitals, 200 clinics and 72 nursing homes, with one or more facilities in all 50 states. It employes about 150,000 personnel. There are major research and teaching programs for physicians and for allied health personnel. VA institutions are affiliated with about 80 medical schools, and about half of the 5,000 full-time VA doctors hold academic appointments.

The passage of Public Law 89-785 in November 1966 gave the VA explicit authority to share facilities with other health institutions, thus increasing the cooperative role of the VA.

The following types of patients are eligible for care in VA hospitals, which are scattered throughout the U.S.:

1. Those requiring treatment for military service-connected disabilities
2. Those requiring treatment for non-service-connected conditions who were either discharged from military service for a disability incurred or aggravated in the line of duty, or who have a compensable service-connected disability
3. Other veterans with wartime service who require treatment for non-service-connected conditions, if they are not able to pay for private hospital care. They must indicate on an affidavit that they are unable to pay for hospital care and include a statement of their assets.
4. Military personnel transferred from military hospitals to continue treatment, who are in the process of being discharged from the armed forces

About 70 percent of VA patients are below the poverty level.

Public Health Service (USPHS). Types of persons treated by USPHS hospitals:

a. American Merchant Seamen
b. Personnel of the U.S. Coast Guard, Coast and Geodetic Survey and their dependents
c. American Indians and Alaskan Eskimos
d. Federal employees injured on duty
e. Persons addicted to narcotic drugs
f. Other

State

Long Term. Every state operates one or more state hospitals emphasizing institutional care of the mentally ill, the retarded, and tuberculosis patients. They are run by departments, boards, or administrative agencies of state governments, such as departments of health or welfare. There are also state schools for the blind, deaf, and mentally deficient, and infirmaries or hospitals connected with state reformatories and prisons. Residents of the state for a certain period of time who are unable to pay for care on a private basis are eligible. Admission to mental hospitals can be a voluntary decision on the part of the patient, or, more frequently, an involuntary commitment by a court on the recommendation of a court-appointed board of examiners, which considers petitions from the patient's family and testimony of psychiatrists in a commitment hearing.

Short Term. Primarily acute care general hospitals controlled by state medical schools as a primary source of patients for educating students, such as the University Hospital in Ann Arbor, Michigan, of the University of Michigan Medical School.

Local

District. These are similar to school, sanitary, water, etc., districts. They are political subdivisions set up for the purpose of maintaining a hospital with the power to tax the population in the district. They are governed by a board of directors which is elected by district residents. As such, they are independent of city, county, or state government. This is not a common form of organization except in a few states, e.g., California.

County. These hospitals are run by the county board of supervisors. They include the large urban hospitals for the indigent, like Cook County Hospital in Chicago. They also include many smaller, rural hospitals which care for both private patients and indigent patients.

City-County. Controlled jointly by municipal and county governments, often for indigent patients.

City. Owned by municipal government and managed by an appointed board of citizens. They include hospitals primarily for the indigent and hospitals for both indigent and paying patients.

Voluntary ("Voluntary" and "nonprofit" are usually used interchangeably.)

Church. A number of religious groups own, operate, or own and operate hospitals. The Roman Catholic Church is foremost of these groups in terms of number of hospitals.

Roman Catholic hospitals are owned and operated by over 100 different sisterhoods (religious orders, or communities of women bound together within the Church by vows of poverty, chastity, and obedience). Most religious orders are expected to be self-sufficient and are relatively independent of each other; however, all orders must abide by the canon laws of the Church. The Mother Superior (sometimes Mother General or Mother Provincial) of the order is usually president of the hospital governing board. A sister usually administers the hospital (although this is changing) and sisters work in a variety of capacities within the hospital, although they are usually only a small fraction of the hospital's total work force. (There are brotherhoods which run hospitals as well, e.g., The Alexian Brothers.)

Other Religious Groups. Over a dozen different Protestant denominations own, operate, or own and operate hospitals. Jewish hospitals are not owned or controlled by religious organizations. Instead, they are independent community hospitals supported by the Jewish community.

Community Hospitals. These are independent, nonprofit hospital corporations or associations composed of public-spirited citizens who are interested in providing hospital care for their community and who organized solely for that purpose. These hospitals, governed by nonprofit associations or corporations which are usually open to any interested citizen, require a small yearly contribution, and can have up to several thousand members, usually meet once a year for the purpose of electing new members of the hospital board of trustees or directors. The board typically has 5 to 15 members, meets monthly, has by-laws, and elects its own officers. The board is subdivided into various commitees: executive, finance, fund-raising, etc. The executive committee typically meets weekly, appoints the administrator, and approves the appointments of physicians to the hospital medical staff. The administrator, in turn, appoints department heads and is in charge of the day-to-day operation of the hospital. There are perhaps as many variations on this theme as there are community hospitals.

Other. A number of hospitals are run by industrial corporations for their employees (railroads, logging) and by unions for their members. The Shriners (the Ancient Arabic Order of Nobles of the Mystic Shrine of North America) own and operate a number of hospitals for crippled children under the age of 14 who are unable to pay their full costs and who have a possibility of cure or rehabilitation to self-sufficiency.

Cooperative Hospitals. These are controlled by the users of health services, and provide comprehensive care, require prepayment by members, and utilize group medical practice. These include the Group Health Association of Washington, D.C., the Group Health Cooperative of Puget Sound, and the Kaiser Foundation.

Proprietary (synonymous with for-profit). Hospitals have traditionally been owned by one physician (*individual owner*) or a group of physicians (as a *partnership* or *corporation*), who usually use these hospitals for the care of their own patients. A recent development is corporations which own a *chain* of hospitals, nursing homes, and/or other health facilities whose stock is sold to the public. These are called *investor-owned* hospital corporations.

Osteopathic Hospitals. (See section on Osteopathy). Osteopathic hospitals are those staffed by Doctors of Osteopathy and are either of the nonprofit community or proprietary types. They are mostly general hospitals.

Hospitals by Type of Patient Treated

a. General Medical and Surgical (General Hospitals)
b. Hospital Unit of an Institution (Prison Hospital, College Infirmary)
c. Psychiatric
d. Tuberculosis
e. Narcotic Addiction, Addictive Diseases
f. Geriatric
g. Maternity
h. Eye, Ear, Nose and Throat
i. Physical Rehabilitation
j. Orthopedic
k. Chronic and Convalescent
l. Institutions for Mental Retardation
m. Epilepsy
n. Alcoholism
o. Other
p. Children's Hospitals, including: General; Unit of an Institution; Psychiatric; Tuberculosis; Eye, Ear, Nose and Throat; Physical Rehabilitation; Orthopedic; Chronic and Convalescent; Other.

**Patient Payment Status and
Types of Accommodation**

Patient Status[3]

a. *Self-Pay* patients pay their own hospital bill without recourse to insurance benefits.
b. *Third Party Paid* patients have part or all of their care paid for by insurance. (Third party to the patient and the practitioner).
c. *Medically Indigent* patients are those who have enough income to live on but are unable to meet the costs of medical care.
d. *Indigent Patients* do not have enough money to live on. Indigent patients are sometimes called poor patients, charity patients, service patients, or ward patients.

Types of Accommodation—*Private, Semi-Private,* and *Ward Patients*
This distinction refers to the type of room the patient occupies in the hospital.

a. A *private patient* occupies a room by himself.

---

[3]The words "case" and "patient" are used synonymously.

b. A *semi-private patient* usually occupies a room with one to three other people (or beds).

c. A *ward patient* occupies a room with three or more other people (or beds). *Private* and *ward* also refer to different physician-patient arrangements. Private patients have their own doctor who they pay for services rendered. Ward (or service or charity) patients are cared for by the doctors in charge of the unit, often including interns and residents, and are supervised by staff physicians.[4]

Teaching Hospitals

Although definitions vary, teaching hospital usually refers to the existence of an approved physician *internship* and/or *residency* program in the hospital. It can also refer to the clinical teaching of medical students in the hospital (medical school affiliation). Medical school affiliation may be by agreement or by ownership, the medical school owning and operating the hospital (for example, the University of Chicago clinics). Hospitals may also be involved in teaching student nurses and other types of personnel. *House staff* refers to both interns and residents combined, as distinct from the *full-time staff* who spend their full working time in the hospital and often may be paid by the hospital or medical school (again, definitions vary), and as distinct from the visiting staff, who are in private practice earning their livelihood through charges to patients.

Frequently Used Hospital Statistics[5]

Patient Days (Patient Bed Days). The total number of inpatient days of care given in a specified time period. For example, if there were 50 patients in the hospital for each day for 10 days this would be 500 patient days for this time period.

Hospital Beds. The average number of beds, cribs, and pediatric bassinets (excluding bassinets for newborn babies) regularly maintained (set up and staffed for use) for inpatients during a period of time (usually a year).

Bassinets. Bassinets, incubators, and isolators for newborn babies in a nursery.

Admissions. Number of patients accepted for inpatient service in a period of time (excluding births).

Discharges and Deaths. Number of inpatients leaving the hospital in a period of time. This usually excludes newborn babies.

Census (Average Daily Census). Number of inpatients receiving care on an average day (excluding newborns). This is usually calculated by counting the number of patients in the hospital every midnight (*midnight census*).

---

[4] See American Association of Medical Record Librarians, *Glossary of Hospital Terms*, (Chicago: The Association, 1969).

[5] American Hospital Association, The Guide Issue, *JAHA*, yearly.

Occupancy. The ratio of census to beds, usually as a percentage of beds in use.

Average Length of Stay (ALOS). Average stay, in days, of inpatients in a given time period. This can be calculated by dividing the number of patient days by either the number of admissions or the number of discharges and deaths.

Available Bed Days. The average number of beds available for use times the number of days in a given time period. Thus, a 100-bed hospital would have 36,500 available bed days per year.

Staffing Ratio. The total number of hospital employees (full-time equivalents) divided by the average daily census.

Per Diem Cost, Cost Per Patient Day. The cost of running the hospital divided by the number of patient days in that time period. Various adjustments or corrections in the cost figures are sometimes made in order to compare hospitals.

Inpatients and Outpatients. Outpatients can also be called *ambulatory* patients or *clinic* patients. Sometimes clinic patients refers to medically indigent patients who use the clinics and associated inpatient ward services. In other hospitals the clinics may be open to both paying and indigent ambulatory patients.

Waiting List. An ordered list of patients awaiting admission to the hospital. The number of patients on that list.

Some Other Definitions

Short-Term and Long-Term Hospitals. These differ according to the average length of stay of the inpatients. According to the American Hospital Association's definition, in short-term hospitals over 50 percent of all patients admitted stay less than 30 days.

Hospital Service Charge (Per Diem Charge). The basic price per day for inpatient care, usually including food, basic nursing care, administrative overhead, use of the facility: those services used by all patients. *Ancillary Charges* are for special diagnostic and treatment services, such as lab tests, X-rays, operating room, etc.

The medical staff in all but the smallest hospitals is divided by specialty, for example surgery medicine, obstetrics gynecology, psychiatry, general practice etc.[6] Each of these services or departments has a chief of services and a more or less formally structured organization with meetings, responsibilities, and policies. These specialty groupings may be associated with separate groups of inpatient beds reserved for the appropriate patients. For example, beds will be set aside solely for the use of obstetrical patients and this unit will be associated

---

[6]For specialties see the section on *Physicians* under *Health Manpower.*

with the obstetrical department of the medical staff. Other specialties may or may not have beds especially designated for their patients. If not their patients would be mixed together with those under the care of other specialists.

3. HOSPITALS (2)

The General Hospital:
Its Internal Characteristics

The Medical Staff. The medical staff consists primarily of physicians and may include dentists, psychologists, podiatrists, etc. For a doctor to be *on the staff* of a hospital, he must have *hospital privileges* or *hospital admitting privileges.*

An *open staff* is one where any licensed physician may admit his private patient to the hospital and care for him there. Although this used to be widespread, it is now very rare.

A *closed staff* means that only those physicians whose applications for staff membership have been reviewed and approved by the hospital's governing body (board of trustees) may admit and care for patients. This is now the customary arrangement.

Usually a physician who desires to be on the staff of the hospital makes out a written application. This application is reviewed by a credentials' committee of the medical staff, which checks to see if he is duly licensed to practice medicine. This committee of staff doctors makes an advisory recommendation to the board of trustees, which has the final legal authority to specify staff membership.[7]

Many hospitals have a number of different classifications of medical staff, which can include the following:

a. *active staff*–the regular membership
b. *associate*–junior membership
c. *consulting*–doctor can consult but not admit
d. *courtesy*–for a doctor who only occasionally uses the hospital
e. *emeritus*–for doctors retired from the active staff
f. *house staff*–interns and residents
g. *honorary*–for noted doctors not heavily involved in the hospital

Usually staff appointments are renewable yearly. In exchange for the privilege of admitting patients to the hospital, staff physicians are usually asked to give some of their time in service to the hospital, often in the form of

---

[7]Again, it is important to remember that there are endless variations on these ways of doing things. What follows can be viewed as typical arrangements.

committee membership, chief of services, teaching, research, etc. The amount of this service varies substantially with the hospital.

The *Medical Staff By-Laws* are rules and regulations which govern the behavior of physicians on the hospital's staff. These by-laws are approved by the governing body of the hospital, with the advice of the medical staff. These by-laws vary from hospital to hospital, but they generally include the following:

1. *Statement of Purpose:* To insure quality of care, to maintain staff self-government and educational standards.
2. *Statement Concerning Membership:* Qualifications, ethical conduct, terms of appointment, procedure for appointment and termination, appeal procedure.
3. *Descriptive Outline of the Medical Staff Organization:* Categories of membership, listing and description of clinical departments.
4. *Statement Concerning Medical Staff Functions:* To be accomplished through medical staff committees which are likely to include (a) executive, (b) credentials, (c) joint conference, (d) accreditation, (e) medical records, tissue, and audit reviews, (f) utilization, (g) infections, (h) pharmacy, (i) other.
5. *Statement of Delineation of Privileges:* Saying what range of patients and treatments each physician may care for and use.
6. *Statement about Staff Meetings:* Including (a) annual meeting, (b) regular departmental, (c) special, (d) attendance records, (e) rules of order, and (f) agenda.
7. *Rules and Regulations:* For (a) keeping accurate and complete medical records, (b) insuring that tissue removed by operation is sent to the laboratory, (c) insuring routine physical examination of all patients on admission and the recording of a pre-operative diagnosis before surgery, (d) insuring that surgical patients give consent to the operation, (e) insuring consultations on special cases, and (f) insuring that physician orders are written and signed.

The staff usually has an overall president and/or chief of staff. The staff is usually subdivided by department (medicine, surgery, pediatrics, obstetrics, gynecology, etc.), each with a chief of service. There may also be a director of medical education.

These positions may be appointed by the governing body or elected by the medical staff or some combination. They may be salaried in full, in part, or not at all. They may have an office in the hospital or may not.

Medical Staff Committees: Some Important Examples

Executive Committee consists of the chiefs of service, elected members of the staff, and other officers, and is the senior decision-making body of the medical staff.

Joint Conference Committee includes officers of the medical staff and members of the governing board for the purpose of maintaining communications between board and staff. Not all hospitals have this committee.

Credentials Committee reviews applications for staff membership.

Utilization Review Committee reviews patient records to insure that it is necessary for patients to be in the hospital. Having such a committee is a requirement for participation in Medicare.

Tissue Committee reviews surgical specimens to see if the tissue was diseased or not. It is presumed to be a check on surgical performance.

Medical Records, Infection, and Pharmacy Committees review performance in these areas of the hospital in connection with medical staff activities.

The extent of committees, full-time chiefs of staff, and formalized medical staff rules depends on the size of the hospital. Larger hospitals tend to be more structured and formalized.

The Medical Record. The medical record is the written record of the patient's progress. Each patient seen in a hospital and in a doctor's private office has a record. When the patient is in the hospital, this record is kept at the nursing station and is also referred to as the *patient's chart.* When the patient is not in the hospital, the chart becomes the medical record and is stored in the Medical Records Department.

The medical record usually includes several separate sections; among them are the following:

a. *admissions form*—patient's name, age, sex, address, attending physician, admission diagnosis, etc.
b. *past history*—relevant family, mental, and personal history; previous illnesses and hospitalizations; allergies
c. *system history*—previous problems associated with different parts of the body
d. *physical examination*—present condition of different parts of the body
e. *summary sheet*—chief complaint, present illness, significant findings, diagnostic impression, and suggested program
f. *daily record of temperature, pulse and respiration (TPR)*—weight, food, treatment, and medication
g. *laboratory data*—laboratory test results
h. *treatment record*—doctor's orders, and his required signature; description of operation and other procedures
i. *nurse's notes*—observations of patient's behavior and condition
j. *discharge note*—disposition (i.e., next steps in treatment), discharge summary of hospitalization, discharge diagnosis, and physician's signature
k. *other special reports*—e.g., autopsy report

The Problem-Oriented Medical Record, recently developed by

Dr. Lawrence L. Weed,[8] is a reorganization of the contents of the medical record. It changes the focus from the admitting diagnosis to a numbered list of all the patient's problems (active and inactive). By so doing, it attempts to avoid guessing at initial diagnoses. Progress toward the resolution of each of these problems is pursued as the focus of the patient's record. Dr. Weed argues that this form of record is better for teaching students and compels attention to the full range of the patient's problems.

Miscellaneous Hospital Terminology

Emergency Admission, emergency surgery must be cared for immediately, in contrast to an *elective admission* (elective surgery) which may be delayed without harm to the patient.

Rounds. "To make rounds" constitutes a physician's visit to the bedsides of his hospitalized patients to note their progress.

Ward Rounds, Teaching Rounds. The teaching physician's bedside review of patients for the purpose of supervising and instructing house staff and medical students (*bedside teaching*).

Grand Rounds. In a hospital, the (usually) weekly description, review, and discussion of a patient (*presentation of a case*), in an auditorium, to all the medical staff of the hospital for the purpose of education.

Clinico-Pathological Conference (CPC). The physical examination and diagnostic test results are described before the full medical staff; an expert then analyzes these findings and attempts a diagnosis. Then the pathologist reports his diagnosis, based on tissue examination.

A *referral* is when one doctor sends a patient to another doctor who specializes in the appropriate area. In doing so, the referring doctor hands over primary responsibility for the patient to that specialist. A *consultation* consists of seeking advice from a specialist (a consultant) without relinquishing primary responsibility for the patient.

References

"Hospital Accreditation References," 1964 edition, American Hospital Association, Chicago, Illinois, 1964.

"General Principles of Medical Staff Organization," American Medical Association, Chicago, Illinois, December 1964.

C. Wesley Eisele (editor), *The Medical Staff in the Modern Hospital,* (New York: McGraw-Hill, 1967).

"Model Medical Staff By-Laws, Rules and Regulations," Joint Commission on Accreditation of Hospitals, Chicago, Illinois, 1964.

Milton Roemer and Jay W. Friedman, *Doctors in Hospitals,* (Baltimore, Md.: The Johns Hopkins Press, 1971).

---

[8]Lawrence L. Weed, M.D., Medical Records, *Medical Education and Patient Care,* (The Press of Case Western Reserve University; distributed by Year Book Medical Publishers, Chicago, Illinois).

T.R. Ponton, *The Medical Staff in the Hospital,* (Chicago, Illinois: The Physicians Record Company, 1953).

4. HOSPITAL DEPARTMENTS AND SERVICES

Hospitals are often organized in two different ways simultaneously. The first way the hospital is organized is that patients are grouped together by specialty in wards, floors or nursing units. For example the hospitals' patients and doctors may be grouped into medical, surgical, pediatric and other specialties. In addition to these inpatient groupings there are groupings of ambulatory patients which may include an emergency unit and various outpatient clinics.

Secondly hospital personnel are grouped into departments such as nursing, dietary, laboratory etc. These departments provide services to all patients who need them. The section that follows will primarily focus on this second way in which hospitals are organized.

This distinction becomes confusing for such units as radiology, laboratories, anesthesiology, physical medicine etc. which include both specialized physicians and other hospital personnel.

The words *department* and *services* are used differently in different hospitals.

Sometimes *services* refers to separate groupings of patients, some personnel, and doctors: for example, surgical, medical, obstetrical, emergency, private, or outpatient services. Most other groupings of hospital personnel would be called *departments,* for example, the X-ray, nursing, and dietary departments.

Sometimes *services* is defined to include personnel who provide services directly to patients: for example, the nursing and dietary services and the maintenance department. Sometimes they are all referred to as *departments*: for example, the surgical department. Sometimes several departments or services are administratively grouped together to form *divisions.*

Excluding medical staff, the departments of the hospital can be grouped under Nursing Services, Ancillary Services, Administration and Support Services.[9] The overall, day-to-day responsibility for the performance of these services lies with the administrator, his associates, and assistants who, in turn, answer to the hospital's governing board. The administrator also may be called *matron* (archaic), *superintendent* (now rare), *general director,* or *president.* Some hospitals have a president, who is concerned with long-term planning, community relations, board of trustees relationships, etc., and an executive vice president, who is responsible for the day-to-day internal management of the hospital. One example of the organization of a large community general hospital is shown in Table 1-1. There are probably as many variations in organization as

[9]For descriptions of types of personnel and their education, see the section on "Health Manpower."

Table 1-1.   An Example of an Organization Chart for a Large Community General Hospital*

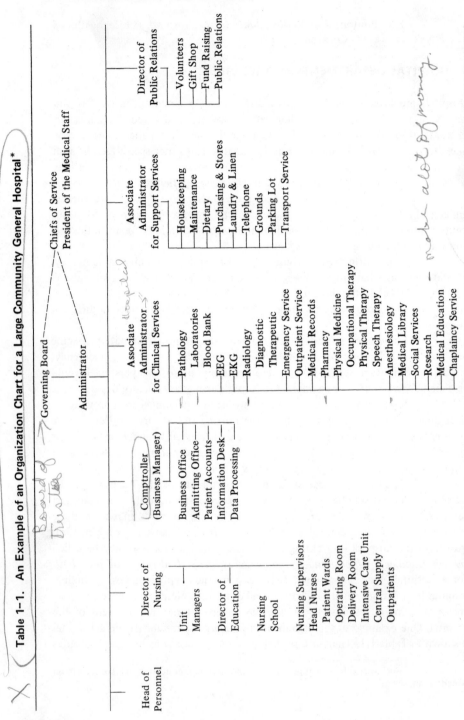

*The internal organization of the medical staff is not shown.

there are hospitals, with respect to which services are offered, how they are grouped, and where they are located within the hospital.

Nursing Services (Department of Nursing, Division of Nursing)

The *Nursing Department* is the single largest component of the hospital. It includes a *director of nursing,* responsible for the whole department; *nursing supervisors,* responsible for several nursing units, each of which is run by a *head nurse;* other nursing personnel on the *nursing unit* (*patient floor* and *ward* are sometimes used to refer to groups of patient rooms in the same place).

Nursing units are often divided up by medical specialty, often including medical, surgical, obstetrical, pediatric, and psychiatric units. There may also be separate units for infectious diseases, *intensive care units* (ICU), and *coronary care units* (CCU). The head nurse directs a group of nursing personnel, including professional nurses (RNs), practical nurses (LPNs), nursing aides, and male orderlies. There is usually a *ward clerk* who copes with the paperwork at the nursing station, where the medical records and medications are kept. There also may be student nurses gaining practical experience and a *unit manager* who carries out a variety of managerial activities, thereby freeing nursing personnel for the care of patients.

Nursing is responsibility for the care of patients on a 24-hour basis. In order to maintain 24-hour coverage, seven days a week, there are three daily nursing shifts, usually a day shift, 7 A.M. to 3 P.M.; an evening shift, 3 P.M. to 11 P.M.; and a night shift, 11 P.M. to 7 A.M.

Other nursing service functions may include the general supervision of the *operating suite,* which consists of *operating rooms* (OR), storage, and associated space such as the *recovery room,* where patients stay immediately after the operation, under close supervision, before returning to their bed on the nursing unit. For obstetrical patients there are *labor rooms, delivery rooms,* and a *newborn nursery* with bassinets for the newborn babies. Maintenance of special cleanliness is vital in all these units and elaborate precautions are taken to prevent infections.

Nursing may include *Central Supply* (also called Central Medical and Surgical Supply, Central Sterile Supply), which washes, packages, and sterilizes (autoclaves) equipment, instruments, gowns, bandages, dressings, etc., primarily for the operating rooms, but also for all parts of the hospital where sterile materials are required. Central Supply may also be responsible for distribution of intravenous solutions (*I-V* fluids, to be injected in patients' veins).

Nursing education may include a hospital school of nursing (a *diploma school*) and *inservice nursing education.* Hospitals which do not have a school of nursing may provide clinical education for nursing students from nearby junior colleges, colleges, or universities for professional nurses (RNs) and for schools for practical nurses.

Ancillary Services   *Review*
Non Renewed.

also mark page 18

Clinical Services (Medical Services).   A number of medical services are hospital-based and may have physical space and hospital personnel working in it. These include:[10]

Anesthesiology. This is a specialty of medicine concerned with the administration of local and general anesthetics, primarily in connection with surgery. This department may include *anesthesiologists* (who are physicians) and/or *nurse-anesthetists,* both of whom administer anesthesia.

Radiology. This department is directed by a *radiologist* (who is a physician), using *X-rays* (or Roentgen rays) for the diagnosis (*diagnostic radiology*) and treatment (*radiation therapy*) of disease. The Department of Nuclear Medicine is sometimes associated with the Radiology Department. *Nuclear medicine* uses radioactive isotopes for the diagnosis and treatment of disease.

The Radiology Department requires a substantial amount of costly equipment and a physical space constructed so as to minimize the hazard of unwanted radiation exposure. A *radiographic technologist* (X-ray technician), who has a required high school education plus two years of training, takes the X-rays, which are then "read," or interpreted by the radiologist.

Pathology (Laboratories, Labs). The hospital laboratories provide examination and analysis of tests on human tissue, bone, and excretions to aid in the diagnosis and treatment of patients. This is usually under the supervision of the hospital's pathologist-in-chief and, in a very large hospital, may include as many as 60 different sub-departments which do special types of analysis and related research. Major subcomponents include:

1. *The clinical laboratory,* which performs tests on blood, urine, bacteria, parasites, etc. Includes *hematology* (the study of blood); *biochemistry* (including the use of automatic analyzers); *bacteriology* (growth and identification of bacteria); *seriology* (antigen-antibody reactions, including the detection of syphilitic infections); *histology* (preparation of tissue removed during surgery); *cytology* (preparation of body fluids to detect cell changes, such as those related to cancer).
2. *The anatomical laboratory* examines tissue both with the microscope and without (gross anatomy). *Autopsies* are performed here to determine the cause of death and a *morgue* for the dead is maintained.

Physical Medicine (Physiatry, Physical and Rehabilitative Medicine). Physiatry, Physical, and Rehabilitative Medicine (physical medicine, for short)

---

[10]Hospital-based physicians working full time within the hospital, particularly radiologists, anesthesiologists, pathologists, physiatrists, and emergency doctors may be paid in a number of different ways, including: (a) a salary from the hospital; (b) by directly billing patients for their services; (c) by a percentage of their department's gross income; (d) by a percentage of their department's net income; (e) a combination of these.

are the same. Physical medicine is a specialty of medicine involved with the diagnosis and treatment of the disabled, convalescent, and physically handicapped patient, using heat, cold, exercise, water, etc., for therapy. *Physical therapists* assist the *physiatrist* (a medical doctor) in these tasks.

This department may also include *occupational therapy* and *speech therapy*. Occupational therapists help handicapped patients learn job-related skills and activities of daily living. Speech therapists help patients overcome speech problems. There are also corrective therapists, music therapists, and recreational therapists.

Outpatient Department (OPD). This department provides care for the nonemergency ambulatory patient, as contrasted with inpatient care. The department may be divided into numerous specialty clinics and may be staffed separately by doctors, nurses, clerks, etc.

Emergency Service (Emergency Room [ER] , Emergency Department, Casualty Ward, Emergency Ward [EW] . . . This department provides immediate care around the clock for acutely ill patients coming to the hospital, although many of the patients using this service may not be acutely ill. There are a growing number of physicians who specialize in emergency medicine. Nurses, clerks, and other personnel may be assigned to this service. The hospital also may have an ambulance service.

Dental Service. This department provides dental care for ambulatory patients and sometimes for inpatients. The *dental staff* of the hospital, although smaller, is organized as part of the hospital's medical staff.

**Some Other Professional and
Therapeutic Services**

The Pharmacy. This service usually purchases drugs and medications, maintains its supply, fills requisitions for the nursing *floor stock,* and fills prescriptions for individual patients. This department is run by the chief pharmacist; a drug and therapeutics committee provides a link with the medical staff. The hospital may maintain a *formulary,* which lists drugs that the medical staff finds acceptable for use in the hospital. It may list drugs by their generic names and permit the pharmacist to substitute between clinically similar drugs. This lowers the drug inventory and lowers the cost of drugs by allowing the pharmacist to purchase in bulk and to use low-cost generic name drugs.

The Blood Bank. This service maintains a supply of blood and blood derivatives such as plasma, for use in the hospital. In large hospitals there may be *organ banks* (e.g., an eye bank) which maintain a supply of human tissue and bone for replacement in other patients.

Electroencephalography (EEG). The EEG technician uses a machine (the electroencephalograph) to record the patient's brain waves with the use of electrodes attached to the patient's head. The recordings usually are interpreted by a physician to detect brain damage.

Electrocardiography (EKG, ECG). The EKG (or ECG) technician uses machinery to record the electrical impulses produced by the heart muscles. These recordings are interpreted by a physician (often a cardiologist) to detect heart disease.

Inhalation Therapy. The inhalation therapist administers oxygen and therapeutic gas and mist inhalations to patients, at the direction of the patients' physicians, outside of the operating room.

Renal Dialysis (Kidney Dialysis). The use of an artificial kidney machine.

Audiology (Audiologist, Speech Pathologist). The diagnosis and treatment of speech language problems.

Family Planning (birth control) services.

Home Care (Hospital-Based Home Care, Organized Home Care Program) provides care by doctors, nurses, social workers, therapists, etc., in the patient's home.

The Medical Records Department maintains, stores, and retrieves patient records and associated patient care statistics. A numbering system is maintained for each patient and an index of patient names and record numbers is maintained to facilitate retrieval. Records are also indexed by disease, operation, and physician responsible for the patient. The records must be complete, signed by the doctor(s) responsible for the patient, and kept confidential so that only authorized personnel may see them. The *medical records librarian* in charge of this department supervises the file clerks, medical transcriptionists, and medical record technicians working in this department.

The Medical Library and the medical librarian in charge of it are not to be confused with the Medical Records Department and the medical record librarian (above). The Medical Library maintains scientific books and journals for the use of the medical staff and sometimes for other professional personnel.

Chaplaincy Service provides pastoral care or religious counsel for patients.

Social Service (Medical and Psychiatric Social Work) focuses on the social, economic, and environmental factors influencing the patient's condition. Knowledge of community resources is used to reduce the environmental and emotional obstacles to recovery, including financial support, post-hospital care (*discharge planning*), and working with the patient's family. Social Service often works very closely with psychiatry (psychiatric social work).

Dietary Services (the kitchen, inpatient food service cafeteria, food storage and purchasing, catering for special events, educational programs for dieticians, special diet kitchen, etc.). The Dietary Services Department may be headed by a *chief dietician* or a *food service manager,* or both. The education of dieticians emphasizes nutrition, the preparation of special diets, and the relationship between food and health. The background and education of food service managers emphasizes the production and management aspects of food preparation. A substantial number of patients may be on special diets (salt free, low fat, etc.) which must be prepared.

Administration

In addition to the administrator, his assistants, and associates, the administration of the hospital may include an *industrial engineer,* a *Data Processing Department* if the hospital has computer facilities, an *Employees' Health Clinic,* a front *Information Desk,* and other departments, some of which are described below.

Public Relations Department (PR). There may be a PR department to provide information about the hospital to the public, patients, and the press.

The Personnel Department recruits, interviews, and screens applicants for hospital positions and maintains salary scales. It keeps records of present and past hospital employees, orients new employees to the hospital, and maintains a position control system so that the complement of hospital jobs cannot be increased without approval of the administration. Personnel can perform many other functions, including *labor relations,* particularly if hospital personnel are unionized.

Fund-Raising may be a temporary or permanent department which solicits gifts and donations to the hospital, often in connection with the construction of new facilities.

Admissions (Admitting Office, Admitting Department) schedules patients for admission, keeps a waiting list, and a list of empty beds. The admissions personnel may assign patients to beds, and collect initial nonmedical information about the patient for the patient's record before he goes to his bed. They notify other parts of the hospital when the patient is admitted.

The Business Office produces patient bills, and collects money from patients and third party payers (accounts receivable). It maintains financial records, prepares budgets and cost reports for the hospital, and does the payroll for hospital employees.

Hospital Volunteers (Auxiliaries, Women's Auxiliary) are public-spirited citizens who donate their time to work for the hospital. They may help in a variety of tasks: escorting patients; arranging flowers; preparing bandages; running a gift shop, coffee shop, or thrift shop (which sells second-hand clothing, books, furniture, etc., and is located outside the hospital), with the proceeds donated to the hospital. Teenage girls who volunteer are often called *candy stripers,* because of the color of the uniforms they wear.

Support Services

Housekeeping is responsible for cleaning the hospital, including floors, walls, and window-washing, and trash disposal.

Maintenance and Plant is often responsible for painting, repairs, carpentry, plumbing, the steam plant, electricity, air conditioning, elevators, fire alarm systems, emergency power sources, etc. There may be personnel assigned to maintain the hospital's *grounds* (ground crew), to run the *parking lot, print shop,* etc.

Purchasing and Stores is responsible for ordering supplies and equipment. It receives, stores, and delivers these items to the part of the hospital where they will be used. *Competitive bids* are sent out for high cost items and the hospital may participate with other hospitals in the area in a *joint purchasing program,* which can save money by purchasing in large volume.

Messenger and Transport Service delivers mail, supplies, and sometimes moves patients.

Laundry and Linen collects, sorts, washes, dries, presses, and repairs sheets, towels, gowns, uniforms, etc., for use in the hospital.

Telephone Switchboard receives incoming calls and maintains a *paging system* for reaching doctors in the hospital.

Some hospitals *contract* for services such as laundry, data processing, housekeeping, dietary, and others, with outside companies, or perform these services jointly with other hospitals (*shared services*).

Progressive Patient Care (PPC)

This is a way of dividing hospital patient services according to the severity of illness and the amount of care used by the patients. Hospitals have used all, part, or none of this system. Patient care levels, starting with the most intensive are:

1. *Intensive Care* (Intensive Care Unit; ICU), for severely ill patients needing a great deal of nursing care and close supervision. The severity of illness is similar in coronary care units (CCU), which treat patients with heart attacks.
2. *Intermediate Care,* for moderately ill patients.
3. *Self-Care,* for inpatients who can walk about, use a central dining area, and who can cope with activities of daily living.
4. *Long-Term Care (Extended Care Unit).*
5. *Home Care* (Hospital-based Home Care, Organized Home Care Program; in contrast to a doctor's home visit), the organized provision of care in the patient's home by nurses, therapists, social workers, physicians, etc.

References
Robert M. Sloane and Beverly L. Sloane, *A Guide to Health Facilities Personnel and Management,* (St. Louis: C.V. Mosby Co., 1971).

U.S. Department of Labor, Manpower Administration, *Job Description and Organizational Analysis for Hospitals and Related Health Services.* Revised Edition. (Washington, D.C.: U.S. Government Printing Office, 1971.)

John R. McGibony, *Principles of Hospital Administration,* Second Edition, (New York: G.P. Putnam's Sons, 1969).

Joseph K. Owen, *Modern Concepts of Hospital Administration,* (Philadelphia: W.B. Saunders, Co., 1962).

American Hospital Association, *Cumulative Guide to Hospital Literature,* (Chicago: The American Hospital Association, Quarterly).

The Flow of Work in a Community
General Hospital

Another way to conceptualize the activities in a community general hospital is to track the events associated with a patient's admission, diagnostic work-up, treatment, and discharge. In Table 1-2 this is done for a patient requiring an uncomplicated elective hernia operation. This operation, called a herniorrhaphy, is one of the most frequent reasons for hospital admission and is not considered a complex or particularly difficult operation. As the table shows, even this routine admission requires the coordinated activities of a large number of different people and departments. Not all hospital personnel are directly involved with every patient and, therefore, only some are included in this table. Other patients would call for the involvement of other types of personnel.

Although this general outline is fairly typical, the details will vary from patient to patient and from hospital to hospital.

5. JOINT COMMISSION ON ACCREDITATION OF HOSPITALS (JCAH)

The JCAH has its origin in 1915 when the American College of Surgeons became concerned with the quality of hospital records. The JCAH was formed in 1952 with a governing board consisting of representatives of the American Medical Association (seven seats), the American Hospital Association (seven seats), the American College of Surgeons (three seats), and the American College of Physicians (three seats). Although the JCAH once covered Canadian hospitals, this is now done by the Canadian Council on Accreditation of Hospitals.

A hospital which wishes to be accredited asks the JCAH to inspect it. The JCAH physician-surveyor visits the hospital and makes his report. The hospital can be unaccredited, accredited for one year, or for three years. The JCAH develops standards of acceptable practice and provides advice to hospitals.

In 1966 the JCAH started a separate accreditation for extended care facilities, nursing homes, and domiciliary homes. In so doing, the JCAH board has been expanded to include representatives of the American Association of Homes of the Aging (one seat) and the American Nursing Home Association (one seat). The offices of the JCAH are located in Chicago.

To qualify for accreditation the hospital must have 25 beds or over, and be accepted for registration by the American Hospital Association.

Table 1-2. Part I
The Progress of a Herniorrhaphy Patient Through a Community General Hospital

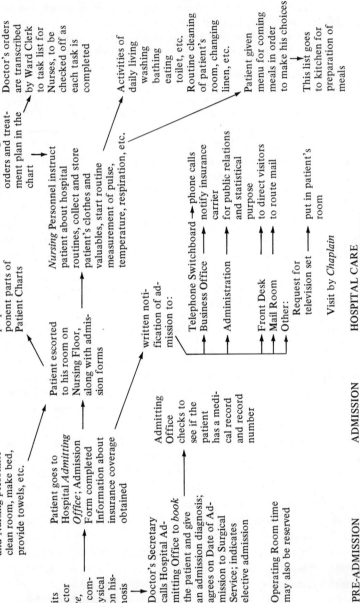

Housekeeping and Nursing personnel clean room, make bed, provide towels, etc.

Ward Clerk prepares component parts of Patient Charts

Doctor writes in his diagnosis orders and treatment plan in the chart

Doctor's orders are transcribed by Ward Clerk to task list for Nurses, to be checked off as each task is completed

Patient escorted to his room on Nursing Floor, along with admission forms

Patient goes to Hospital *Admitting Office;* Admission Form completed Information about insurance coverage obtained

Nursing Personnel instruct patient about hospital routines, collect and store patient's clothes and valuables, start routine measurement of pulse, temperature, respiration, etc.

Activities of daily living
washing
bathing
eating
toilet, etc.
Routine cleaning of patient's room, changing linen, etc.

written notification of admission to:

Admitting Office checks to see if the patient has a medical record and record number

Telephone Switchboard → phone calls
Business Office → notify insurance carrier
Administration → for public relations and statistical purpose

Front Desk → to direct visitors
Mail Room → to route mail
Other:

Request for television set → put in patient's room

Visit by *Chaplain*

Patient given menu for coming meals in order to make his choices

This list goes to kitchen for preparation of meals

Patient visits Private Doctor in his *office,* presenting complaints, physical examination history, diagnosis

Doctor's Secretary calls Hospital Admitting Office to *book* the patient and give an admission diagnosis; agrees on Date of Admission to Surgical Service; indicates elective admission

Operating Room time may also be reserved

PRE-ADMISSION
AMBULATORY CARE

ADMISSION

HOSPITAL CARE
PRE-OPERATIVE CARE

Table 1-2. Part II

delivery of flowers, gifts, mail, newspapers

regulation of *visiting hours* and number of visitors

visit by *chaplain*

hospital volunteer visits (book exchange, patient library, gift cart, etc.)

Visit by *Anesthesiologist* to explain operation, review chart and evaluate patient's condition

On review of these and other findings, the final decision to operate is made by attending doctor → orders pre-operative medication and preparation

Patient signs Operative Consent Form

Patient shaved and cleaned for operation by *Orderly*

Preoperative light diet

Preoperative medication given

Patient transported to *operating room*

Samples of blood and urine taken → sent with order form to *laboratory* for analysis → results reported to Nursing Station and recorded in chart → Forms sent to Business Office for Patient Billing

Patient booked in Radiology Department for Barium Enema

Patient given enema prior to exam → Patient escorted to *Radiology* Department → Examination by Radiology Technician and Radiologist → Patient returns to floor

immediate verbal report to attending doctor

written report for patient record

reading of films taken and storage of X-ray films

Dietician notified of special pre-examination diet

Patient scheduled for *physical therapy* instruction

Physical Therapist visits patient to give instructions to patient on breathing techniques to relieve post-operative pain

Central Supply Room packs and sterilizes instruments for operation

Medication ordered from hospital *Pharmacy* or obtained from Nursing floor stock

Scheduling of Operating Room, if not done before this

Preparation of operating room, cleaning, sterilized linen, and instruments and equipment

PRE-OPERATIVE PERIOD

as a result of the attending doctor's orders

Table 1–2.   Part III
The Progress of a Herniorrhaphy Patient Through a Community General Hospital

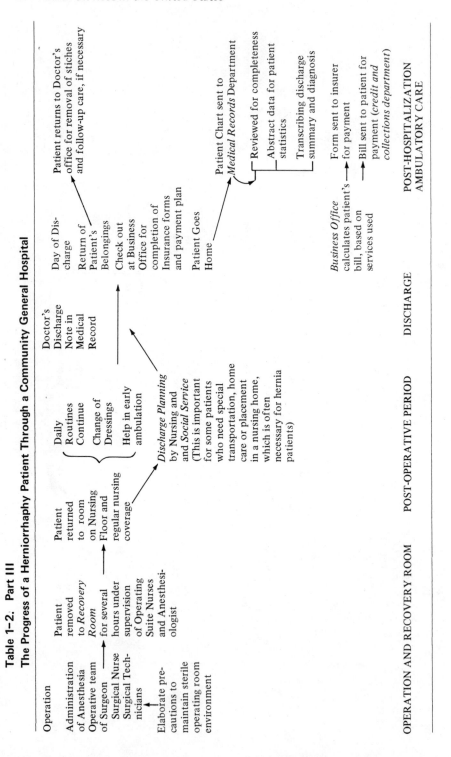

OPERATION AND RECOVERY ROOM	POST-OPERATIVE PERIOD	DISCHARGE	POST-HOSPITALIZATION AMBULATORY CARE
Operation	Patient returned to room on Nursing Floor and regular nursing coverage	Doctor's Discharge Note in Medical Record	Patient returns to Doctor's office for removal of stiches and follow-up care, if necessary
Administration of Anesthesia			
Operative team of Surgeon Surgical Nurse Surgical Technicians	Daily Routines Continue	Day of Discharge	
	Change of Dressings	Return of Patient's Belongings	
Patient removed to *Recovery Room* for several hours under supervision of Operating Suite Nurses and Anesthesiologist	Help in early ambulation	Check out at Business Office for completion of Insurance forms and payment plan	
	Discharge Planning by Nursing and *Social Service* (This is important for some patients who need special transportation, home care or placement in a nursing home, which is often necessary for hernia patients)	Patient Goes Home	Patient Chart sent to *Medical Records* Department
Elaborate precautions to maintain sterile operating room environment			Reviewed for completeness
			Abstract data for patient statistics
			Transcribing discharge summary and diagnosis
		Business Office calculates patient's bill, based on services used	Form sent to insurer for payment
			Bill sent to patient for payment (*credit and collections department*)

6. NURSING HOMES

Prior to 1930 there were very few nursing homes. The Social Security Act of 1935, by making money available to the elderly beneficiaries, encouraged the growth of proprietary boarding and nursing homes and the decline of public alms houses serving the indigent.

Medicare and Medicaid provided further impetus to the growth of nursing homes. All states license nursing homes, not all of which participate in Medicare or Medicaid. In 1966 the JCAH assumed responsibility for the voluntary accreditation of extended care, nursing care, and resident care facilities.

Today almost one in twenty Americans 65 years old and older occupies a bed in a nursing or related home. About 90 percent of nursing home patients are over 65. The majority of nursing homes are proprietary. Nursing homes are licensed by the state and, in addition, are usually certified for participation in Medicare and Medicaid. Prior to the passage of PL 92-603 nursing homes were classified as Skilled Nursing Homes, Extended Care Facilities (ECF), and Intermediate Care Facilities (see Table 1-3).

Table 1-3. Nursing and Related Homes Recognized under Government Programs

Type of Service*	Program	Care Supported	Types of Institutions
Skilled Nursing Home	Medicaid	Primarily long-term skilled nursing	Primarily nursing homes, also special sections of hospitals and in homes for the aged.
Extended Care Facility	Medicare	Post-hospital skilled nursing (100 day limit)	Primarily nursing homes, also extended care facilities and special sections in hospitals
Intermediate Care Facility	Medicaid	Primarily long-term supportive	Homes for the aged, rest homes, supportive care homes, personal care homes, and sections in nursing homes

*These facility categories are not mutually exclusive and the first two categories broadly overlap.
Source: Kenneth Frank, "Government Support of Nursing Home Care," *New England Journal of Medicine*, Sept. 14, 1972, p. 538.

Today the ECF is no longer a distinct classification of facility, but has been merged into the category of Skilled Nurse Facility (SNF, pronounced "Sniff"). In addition to the three levels of SNF, ICF (Intermediate Care Facility), and Residential Facility, the states usually define four levels of nursing home care. The higher the level of care, the greater the care needs of the patient and the higher the level of reimbursement from Medicaid (see Table 1-4).

Table 1-4. Revised Classification of Nursing Homes Recognized under Government Programs since June 1973

Federal Designation of Type of Service	State Designation of Levels of Care*	Paid for by
Skilled Nursing Facility (SNF)	I and II	Medicare and Medicaid
Intermediate Care Facility (ICF)	III	Medicaid
Residential Facility (Rest Home)	IV	

*There are single-level and multi-level facilities

SNFs provide continuous nursing service on a 24-hour basis. Registered nurses, licensed practical nurses, and nursing aides provide services prescribed by the patient's physician. The emphasis is on medical nursing care with restorative therapy, physical therapy, occupational therapy, etc. Medicare and Medicaid pay for care in SNFs. Medicare will pay if

a. the home is certified as a SNF;
b. the patient has spent at least three consecutive days in a hospital and is admitted to the SNF within 14 days after discharge;
c. the patient's physician says the care is needed for the illness for which the patient has been hospitalized;
d. skilled nursing care and rehabilitative services as defined by the Social Security Administration are required by the patient on a daily basis.

Medicare pays for the first twenty days and for part of the next eighty days, if the patient qualifies. A utilization review mechanism is required.

Unlike Medicare, Medicaid program benefits vary from state to state. Medicare does not provide ICF benefits, but Medicaid does.

The intermediate care facility is intended as a less expensive alternative to the skilled nursing home in the same way that the skilled nursing home is intended as a substitute for the more expensive hospital.

Three associations represent nursing homes. The American Nursing Home Association (the largest, representing profit and not-for-profit homes), the American Association of Homes for the Aging (represents only non-profit homes), and the National Council of Health Care Services (large for-profit nursing home chains). In addition, there are 300 national organizations representing the elderly.

Three types of services are offered in nursing homes.

1. *Nursing care:* by RNs and LPNs. Also physical therapy, occupational therapy, dental services, dietary consultations, lab, X-ray services, and a pharmaceutical dispensary
2. *Personal care:* help in walking, getting in and out of bed, bathing, dressing and eating, preparation of special diets prescribed by a physician
3. *Residential care:* room and board in a protective environment and a planned program for the residents' social and spiritual needs

Nursing homes vary according to services provided, from those with extensive nursing and other services (including full-time physicians), personal care homes with and without nursing, domiciliary homes (homes for the aged), and special housing for the aged.[11]

Licensure of *nursing home administrators* (SNFs, ICFs) is mandatory in all states. Licensure requires 15 hours a year of continuing education.

7. OTHER HEALTH SERVICES

Ambulance Services

Emergency ambulance services are provided by police departments, fire departments, volunteer community groups, welfare departments, morticians, hospitals, taxi companies, gasoline service stations and commercial ambulance companies. They use a variety of vehicles, from completely equipped modern ambulances to station wagons and trucks.

Almost half of the country's 13,000 ambulance services (23,300 vehicles) are provided by funeral homes. All states regulate the operation of ambulances except North Dakota (1971).

Clinical (Medical) Laboratories

These laboratories carry out tests on specimens from the human body to detect the presence, absence or extent of disease. They may be physically located in a doctor's office, group practice, hospital, public health agency, or as a privately owned corporation. An independent lab may operate under the direction of a physician or other scientist.

Medicare certifies 2,750 independent labs (independent of attending consulting doctor's office or hospitals).

Dental Laboratories

These laboratories fabricate dentures and other dental appliances; by 1970 there were an estimated 9,000 commercial dental laboratories in the

---

[11] The "aged," the "elderly," "old people," "senior citizens," and "golden age groups" are used interchangeably for people 65 years old and over.

U.S.; 4,400 in dental offices, 700 in federal dental services, and 100 in educational institutions.

There is a Joint Commission on the Accreditation of Dental Laboratories.

Optician Establishments

These establishments compound, fill, and adapt opthalmic prescriptions, products, and accessories: primarily selling eyeglasses.

Tables 1-5– 1-9 provide some basic data on hospitals, nursing homes, and other inpatient services.

Table 1–5. Hospitals and Hospital Beds: Selected Years 1963 through 1970

		General medical and surgical	Specialty				
Year	Total hospitals		Total	Psychiatric	Geriatric and chronic	Tuberculosis	Other[1]
			Facilities				
1970	7,638	6,574	1,064	494	126	108	336
1969	7,845	6,715	1,130	506	189	116	319
1968	7,991	6,539	1,452	494	291	129	538
1967	8,147	6,685	1,462	573	333	169	387
1963	8,183	6,710	1,473	581	211	258	423
			Beds				
1970	1,534,779	1,004,415	530,364	437,969	38,144	19,836	34,415
1969	1,565,908	989,733	576,175	477,309	40,790	20,960	37,116
1968	1,564,444	934,297	630,147	503,042	43,921	25,381	57,803
1967	1,631,101	958,729	672,372	545,913	61,211	33,335	31,913
1963	1,549,952	811,876	738,076	614,104	38,213	50,075	35,685
			Beds per 1,000 population				
1970	7.6	5.0	2.6	2.2	0.2	0.1	0.2
1969	7.8	5.0	2.9	2.4	0.2	0.1	0.2
1968	7.9	4.7	3.2	2.5	0.2	0.1	0.3
1967	8.3	4.9	3.4	2.8	0.3	0.2	0.2
1963	8.3	4.3	4.0	3.3	0.2	0.3	0.2

[1] Includes eye, ear, nose, and throat hospitals; epileptic hospitals; alcoholic hospitals; narcotic hospitals; maternity hospitals; orthopedic hospitals; physical rehabilitation hospitals and other hospitals.

Source: *Health Resources Statistics,* 1971. National Center for Health Statistics, USDHEW, PHS, HSMHA (Rockville, Maryland), February 1972, p. 302.

From: Unpublished data from the National Center for Health Statistics master facility census. National Center for Health Statistics: *Health Resources Statistics,* 1969. PHS Pub. 1509. Public Health Service, U.S. Department of Health, Education and Welfare. Washington. U.S. Government Printing Office, May 1970. U.S. Bureau of the Census: *Current Population Reports.* Series P-25, No. 462, June 1971.

Table 1-6. Ownership of Hospitals: 1970

Ownership	Total Hospitals	General medical and surgical	Specialty Total	Psychiatric	Geriatric and chronic	Tuberculosis	Other[1]
Total	7,638	6,574	1,064	494	126	108	336
Government	2,755	2,198	557	324	71	101	61
Federal	412	375	37	31	1	2	3
State-local	2,343	1,823	520	293	70	99	58
Proprietary	1,034	863	171	80	15	1	75
Nonprofit	3,849	3,513	336	90	40	6	200
Church	930	862	68	15	7	1	45
Other	2,919	2,651	268	75	33	5	155

[1] Includes eye, ear, nose, and throat hospitals; epileptic hospitals, alcoholic hospitals; narcotic hospitals; maternity hospitals; orthopedic hospitals; physical rehabilitation hospitals; and other hospitals.

Source: *Health Resources Statistics,* 1971. National Center for Health Statistics, USDHEW, PHS, HSMHA (Rockville, Maryland), February 1972, p. 309.

From: Unpublished data from the National Center for Health Statistics master facility census.

Table 1-7. Ownership of Nursing Care and Related Homes: 1969

Ownership	Total homes	Nursing care	Personal care homes With nursing	Personal care homes Without nursing	Domiciliary care
			Number of homes		
Total homes	18,910	11,484	3,514	3,792	120
Government	1,390	546	316	506	22
Federal	69	22	18	28	1
State-local	1,321	524	298	478	21
Proprietary	14,470	9,321	2,187	2,879	83
Nonprofit	3,050	1,617	1,011	407	15
Church	1,038	559	383	92	4
Other	2,012	1,058	628	315	11
			Number of beds		
Total beds	943,876	704,217	174,874	63,532	1,253
Government	88,113	57,051	22,809	8,094	159
Federal	3,523	526	2,749	243	5
State-local	84,590	56,525	20,060	7,851	154
Proprietary	629,277	520,615	64,669	43,150	843
Nonprofit	226,486	126,551	87,396	12,288	251
Church	89,255	44,868	41,137	3,204	46
Other	137,231	81,683	46,259	9,084	205

Source: *Health Resources Statistics,* 1971. National Center for Health Statistics, USDHEW, PHS, HSMHA (Rockville, Maryland), February 1972, p. 327.

From: Unpublished data from the National Center for Health Statistics master facility census.

Table 1-8. Inpatient Health Facilities: Selected Years 1963 through 1970

Type of facility	1963	1967	1969	1970
Total facilities	27,171	30,586	31,055	–
Hospitals	8,183	8,147	7,845	7,638
General medical and surgical hospitals	6,710	6,685	6,715	6,574
Specialty hospitals	1,473	1,462	1,130	1,064
Psychiatric	581	573	506	494
Geriatric and chronic	[2]211	333	189	126
Tuberculosis	258	169	116	108
Other[1]	423	387	319	336
Nursing care and related homes	16,701	19,141	[2]18,910	–
Nursing care	8,128	10,636	11,484	–
Personal care home with nursing	4,958	3,853	3,514	–
Personal care home without nursing	2,927	4,396	3,792	–
Domiciliary care	688	256	120	–
Other inpatient health facilities	2,287	3,298	[2] 4,300	–

[1]Includes eye, ear, nose and throat hospitals; epileptic hostipals; alcoholic hospitals; narcotic hospitals; maternity hospitals; orthopedic hospitals; physical rehabilitation hospitals; and other hospitals.

[2]Revised.

Source: *Health Resources Statistics,* 1971. National Center for Health Statistics, USDHEW, PHS, HSMHA (Rockville, Maryland) February 1972, p. 296.

From: Unpublished data from the National Center for Health Statistics master facility census.

8. REGULATION OF HEALTH SERVICES INSTITUTIONS

Regulation, broadly defined, can be classified as *governmental* and *voluntary.* Regulation can be internal or external to the organization. It can be done by professionals collectively, or it can be done by consumers and laymen. It can be achieved through voice or exit[12] (see Table 1-10 and section on "Quality Control").

Health organizations regulate the performance of their personnel through *administrative policies and procedures.* In addition, the professionals who practice in organizational settings abide by collectively defined rules and by-laws, and by *peer review* of performance. Organizations may elect to abide by the recommended policies of external accrediting agencies, such as *voluntary planning groups,* the JCAH, and educational accrediting groups. An important part of professional education is the internalizing of ethical values which enjoin the professional to strive for high ideals of public service and a commitment to excellence. The AMA

[12]Albert O. Hirschman, *Exit Voice and Loyalty* (Cambridge, Mass.: Harvard University Press, 1970).

Table 1-9. Beds in Inpatient Health Facilities: Selected Years 1963 through 1970

Type of facility	Number				Number per 1,000 population			
	1963	1967	1969	1970	1963	1967	1969	1970
Total beds	2,448,512	2,871,655	2,952,784	—	13.1	14.7	14.8	—
Hospitals	1,549,952	1,631,101	1,565,908	1,534,779	8.3	8.3	7.8	7.6
General medical and surgical hospitals.	811,876	958,729	989,733	1,004,415	4.3	4.9	5.0	5.0
Specialty hospitals	738,076	672,372	576,175	530,364	4.0	3.4	2.9	2.6
Psychiatric	614,104	545,913	477,309	437,969	3.3	2.8	2.4	2.2
Geriatric and chronic	38,213	61,211	40,790	38,144	0.2	0.3	0.2	0.2
Tuberculosis	50,074	33,335	20,960	19,836	0.3	0.2	0.1	0.1
Other[1]	35,685	31,913	37,116	34,415	0.2	0.2	0.2	0.2
Nursing care and related homes.	568,560	836,554	[2]943,876	—	3.0	4.3	4.7	—
Nursing care	319,224	584,052	704,217	—	1.7	3.0	3.5	—
Personal care home with nursing	188,306	181,096	174,874	—	1.0	0.9	0.9	—
Personal care home without nursing	48,962	66,787	63,532	—	0.3	0.3	0.3	—
Domiciliary care	12,068	4,619	1,253	—	0.1	0.0	0.0	—
Other inpatient health facilities	330,000	404,000	[3]443,000	—	1.8	2.1	2.2	—

[1]Includes eye, ear, nose, and throat hospitals; epileptic hospitals; alcoholic hospitals; narcotic hospitals; maternity hospitals; orthopedic hospitals; physical rehabilitation hospitals and other hospitals.

[2]Revised estimates.

[3]Estimated.

Source: *Health Resources Statistics,* 1971. National Center for Health Statistics, USDHEW, PHS, HSMHA (Rockville, Maryland), February 1972, p. 297.

From: Unpublished data from the National Center for Health Statistics master facility census. U.S. Bureau of the Census: *Current Population Reports.* Series P-25. Nos. 417, 436, 442, and 462.

Table 1–10.   Typology of Regulation

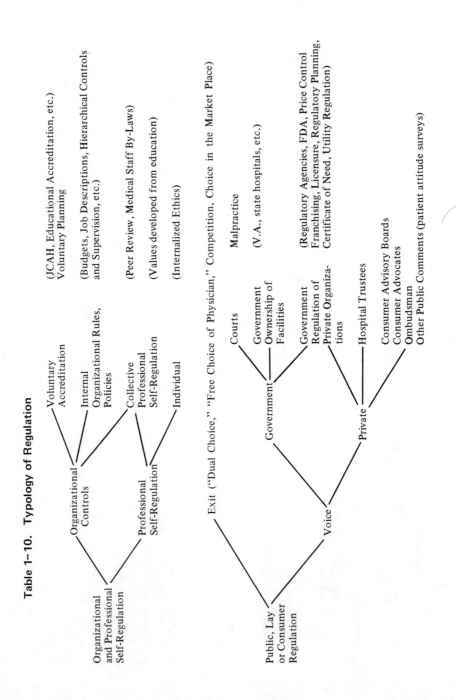

has developed such a Code of Medical Ethics for physicians. To the extent that these ethical ideals are internalized, they are a form of professional self-regulation.

Public, Lay, or Consumer Regulation

The *public* are all people, whether or not they are receiving care.

A *layman* is a nonprofessional; as in "a lay board of trustees."

A *consumer* is a *patient,* a recipient of care, or a purchaser of a health-related product. Public regulation is derived either through "exit," that is, choice in the market place, or "voice," that is, speaking out about their preferences. Part of the aim of public regulations is often to promote and encourage organizational and professional self-regulation.

Exit ("Free choice of physician") refers to the idea that patients should have a choice of physician. *Dual Choice* is usually used in the context of HMO's and PGP's, where the insured person has a choice of either the HMO or insurance coverage which will pay for the non-plan doctor and hospital of his choice.

Voice can be through government or private channels. The former includes redress from *malpractice* through the courts, government ownership and operation of health services, and government regulation of private organizations, some of which are described below. Private channels include (lay) *boards of trustees* which have direct responsibility for the operation of the organization, and *consumer advisory boards* which serve in an advisory capacity. An *ombudsman* is an employee of an organization (public or private) who is responsible for channeling patient complaints and helping resolve problems that arise this way. A *consumer advocate* acts as an ombudsman, but may or may not be employed by a health delivery organization. In addition, public comments may be elicited systematically through *patient attitude surveys,* or may be initiated by patients in an informal way.

The influence of these regulatory mechanisms will vary from organization to organization and there is no consensus as to their relative impact on the delivery of health services.

Government Regulation of Health Institutions is primarily at the state level, with some exceptions at the federal level, such as the *FDA,* and the *Price Control Commission* which regulates allowable price increases.

Licensure. Hospitals, nursing homes, pharmacies, and sometimes other facilities such as clinics are licensed by the state. They are periodically inspected to insure that they meet minimum standards. In addition, health facilities, like non-health-related buildings, are subject to a variety of inspections for *fire safety, building codes, zoning regulations, boiler* and *elevator performance,* etc.

Institutional Licensure is a concept which is nowhere in actual practice. Instead of licensing doctors, nurses, and other professionals who work in an organization, the organization itself would be licensed so that the personnel working within the organization would be exempt from professional licensure. Then, for example, nurses would be allowed to perform tasks in the organization which are ordinarily restricted to physicians. The idea is that there would be more flexibility and substitution with respect to who does what. It would also minimize *blocked mobility,* in other words, the opportunity for an LPN to do the work of an RN, and an RN to do the work of an M.D.

Certificate of Need Laws. About half the states have such laws to the effect that no health facility can spend more than some specified amount (say, $100,000) on a new construction without state approval. The facility must justify to the state agency that the construction is needed and will not duplicate existing facilities (*duplication of services*).

Franchising. The state establishes conditions under which the hospital or other providor may do business. This idea comes from franchising in business.

Utility Regulation proposes that facilities be regulated by a regulatory board or agency, appointed or controlled by the state, which has the power to approve budgets, prices, expansion, profits, and scope of services provided, in the same way that other utilities (such as electrical and telephone companies) are now regulated.

Health Authority. The creation of a single state organization which controls all licensure of facilities and personnel, and regulation of health insurance, and which channels state and federal funds to private health organizations. This follows the model of port and airport authorities.

Regionalization is the concept that health facilities should be responsible for geographically-defined populations and that there should be systematic relationships and referral patterns between different facilities. For example, there might be "front line" clinics for *primary ambulatory care* linked to community hospitals for *secondary care.* The community hospitals would be linked to medical centers or referral hospitals (*tertiary care*) for very specialized care. This example can be shown diagrammatically as follows:

Nursing homes and other facilities could also be included. As such, regionalization is a concept for the flow of patients and location of services, rather than regulation per se. This concept is transformed into regulation via *Regional Planning.* Regional planning originally started on a voluntary basis for hospitals. This has been largely superceded by the Comprehensive Health Planning and Public Health Amendments of 1966 (PL 89-749). This law created *local health planning agencies* called *314-B Agencies* or *B agencies,* and *state-wide health planning agencies* called *314-A Agencies* or *A agencies.* (314-A and 314-B are the relevant paragraphs in PL 89-749.)

The activities of planning agencies include collecting data to measure use and need; soliciting opinions from the public and providers; giving advice to providers; and varying degrees of control through sanctions.

Chapter Two

Health Manpower

1. OVERVIEW

Personnel, Manpower, Professions in the Health Field

Professional, Paraprofessional, Subprofessional, Semiprofessional. The word professional has no consistent or agreed upon meaning. Most occupational groups in the health field aspire to being considered professions. There are a number of components:[1]

1. Formal education and examination are required for membership in the profession.
2. Certification or licensure is required for membership, reflecting community sanction or approval.
3. The existence of regional or national associations.
4. There is a code of ethics.
5. There is a body of systematic scientific knowledge and technical skill required.
6. The members function with a degree of autonomy and authority, under the assumption that they alone have the expertise to make decisions in their area of competence.

Medicine is often considered the occupation which most closely approaches the prototype of a profession.

---

[1] See Ernest Greenwood, "Attributes of a Profession," p. 206 in Sigmund Nosow and William H. Form (editors), *Man, Work, and Society* (New York: Basic Books, 1962) and Eliot Freidson, *Profession of Medicine* (New York: Dodd Mead & Co., 1970).

41

Paraprofessional or *ancillary personnel* refer to those who work alongside a professional; *subprofessional* refers to occupations which are subordinate to other professions; and *semiprofessionals* do not have all the characteristics of a profession.[2] *Allied* health personnel are those who work with doctors; this category usually includes all hospital personnel, but excludes, for example, chiropractors.

Certification and Licensure.   Certification is the recognition that a person meets certain qualifications for an occupation but does not exclude others from working in that occupation. Certification may be done by an independent organization or by the state. Licensure is a recognition of competence by the state, which excludes or limits nonlicensed people from taking up the occupation. State licensure boards are usually made up of members of the occupation being licensed: (pharmacists, physicians, osteopaths, professional and practical nurses, dentists, podiatrists, and optometrists are among those professionals licensed by the state. The other occupations discussed here are usually not.)

The terms technologist, therapist, technician, assistant and aide are now used in no systematic way. The following definitions are suggested:[3]

Technologist
Therapist — This occupation requires education at, or above, the baccalaureate level

Technician
Assistant — Requires education at, or beyond, the two-year college level (the Associate Degree level) after high school

Aide — Requires less than two years beyond high school or on-the-job training

In the sections that follow there will be more space devoted to physicians, dentists, and nurses because these health occupations are most frequently referred to, and their education is often used as a foil or mirror to compare with that of other professional groups.

Health Professions and Occupations

There are over two hundred occupations in the health field and new ones are constantly appearing. Table 2-1 lists some of these occupations. Table 2-2 estimates the total number of personnel within selected health care occupations. Table 2-3 lists those agencies and organizations that accredit educational programs for selected occupations. Table 2-4 diagrammatically shows the

---

[2] Etzioni, Amitai (editor), *The Semi-Professions and Their Organization* (The Free Press, 1961). The ill-defined word *ancillary personnel* is also used here.

[3] *Health Resources Statistics* HEW, HSMHA, February 1972.

number of years of education beyond high school associated with one hundred health occupations.[4]

Needless to say, there is not enough room to describe all these fields; therefore, a small number of them has been selected for description here. We hope our readers will understand that just because this section does not describe groups such as psychiatric art therapists and marine physician assistants (serving U.S. merchant marine sailors at sea), it does not mean that these groups do not have important roles and useful tasks to perform.

Table 2-1. List of Health Occupations

Primary title (1)	*Alternate title*
1. Administration: Health administrator	Health officer or commissioner. Environmental control administrator. Health agency executive director. Health care administrator. Hospital administrator. Medical care administrator. Nursing home administrator. Public health administrator.
Health administrative assistant Health program analyst	Public health analyst. Public health specialist.
Health program representative	Public health advisor. Public health representative.
Health systems analyst 2. Biomedical Engineering: Biomedical engineer	Bioengineer. Medical engineer.
Biomedical engineering technician Biomedical engineering aide	Medical engineering technician.

3. Chiropractic and Naturopathy:
    Chiropractor
    Naturopath
	Doctor of chiropractic.
	Naturopathic physician.

4. Clinical Laboratory Services (*2*): Clinical laboratory scientist (*3*)	Clinical chemist (*3*). Microbiologist (*3*).
Clinical laboratory technologist	Medical laboratory technologist. Medical technologist. Blood banking technologist. Chemistry technologist. Hematology technologist. Microbiology technologist.

---

[4]This table is taken from *Health Careers Guidebook,* United States Department of Labor, Bureau of Employment Security, (Washington, D.C.: U.S. Government Printing Office), a publication giving basic information on these occupations. Also see the annual "Guide Issue" of *Hospitals, Journal of the American Hospital Association* for a listing of approved schools for health occupations.

Primary title *(1)*	Alternate title
Clinical laboartory technician	Medical laboratory technician. Medical technician. Cytotechnician. Cytotechnologist.
Clinical laboratory aide	Laboratory assistant. Certified laboratory assistant. Histologic aide. Histologic technician. Pathology laboratory aide.

5. Dentistry and Allied Services:

Dentist	Endodontist. Oral pathologist. Oral surgeon. Orthodontist. Pedodontist. Periodontist. Prosthodontist. Public health dentist.
Dental hygienist Dental assistant Dental laboratory technician	 Dental laboratory assistant.

6. Dietetic and Nutritional Services:

Dietitian	Administrative dietition. Consultant (public health) dietition. Research dietitian. Teaching dietitian. Therapeutic dietitian.
Nutritionist *(3)*	Public health nutritionist.
Dietary technician	Dietary (food service) assistant. Food service manager. Food service technician.
Dietary aide Food service supervisor	Dietary (food service) worker.

7. Environmental Control *(4)*:

Environmental scientist *(3)*	Sanitary sciences specialist *(3)*. Air pollution meteorologist *(3)*. Environmental control chemist *(3)*. Estuarine oceanographer *(3)*. Ground water hydrologist *(3)*. Health physicist *(3)*. Limnologist *(3)*.
Environmental engineer	Sanitary engineer. Air pollution engineer. Hospital engineer. Industrial hygiene engineer. Public health engineer. Radiological health engineer.
Environmental technologist	Sanitarian.

Primary title (1)	*Alternate title*
	Air pollution specialist.
	Industrial hygienist.
	Radiological health specialist.
Environmental technician	Sanitarian technician.
	Environmental engineering technician.
	Radiological health technician (monitor).
Environmental aide	Sanitarian aide.
	Environmental engineering aide.
	Sewage plant assistant.
	Waterworks assistant.

8. Food and Drug Protective Services:
   Food technologist
   Food and drug inspector
   Food and drug analyst
   Food and drug technician
9. Health Education:

Health educator	Community health educator.
	Public health educator.
	School health coordinator.
	School health educator.

   Health education aide
10. Information and Communication:

Health information specialist	Biomedical communication specialist.
Health science writer	Medical writer.
Health technical writer	Medical technical writer.
	Medical editor.
Medical illustrator	Medical photographer.

11. Library Services:
    Medical librarian
    Medical library assistant

Hospital librarian	Patients' librarian.

12. Mathematical Sciences (*4*):

Mathematician	Biomathematician.
	Demographer.
Statistician	Biostatistician.
	Health statistician.
	Vital record registrar.

13. Medical Records:

Medical record librarian	Medical record specialist.
	Medical record technologist.
Medical record technician	Medical record assistant.
Medical record clerk	Medical record aide.

14. Medicine and Osteopathy:

Physician	Doctor of medicine—M.D.
Osteopathic physician	Doctor of osteopathy—D.O.
M.D. or D.O.	Allergist.
	Anesthesiologist.
	Aviation medicine specialist.

Primary title (1)	Alternate title
	Cardiovascular disease specialist.
	Colon and rectal surgeon (proctologist).
	Dermatologist.
	Forensic pathologist.
	Gastroenterologist.
	General practitioner.
	Gynecologist.
	Internist.
	Manipulative therapy specialist.
	Neurological surgeon.
	Neurologist.
	Occupational medicine specialist.
	Obstetrician.
	Ophthalmologist.
	Orthopedic surgeon.
	Otolaryngologist (otorhinolaryngologist).
	Pathologist.
	Pediatrician (5).
	Physiatrist (physical medicine and rehabilitation specialist).
	Plastic surgeon.
	Preventive medicine specialist.
	Psychiatrist (6).
	Public health physician.
	Pulmonary disease specialist.
	Radiologist (7).
	Surgeon.
	Thoracic surgeon.
	Urologist.
	Intern.
	Resident.
	Fellow.
15. Midwifery:	
Midwife	Lay midwife.
	Nurse midwife (8).
16. Natural Sciences (4):	
Anatomist	Cytologist.
	Embryologist.
	Histologist.
Botanist	
Chemist	Bioanalyst.
	Biochemist.
	Clinical chemist (9).
	Environmental control chemist (10).
Ecologist	
Entomologist	
Epidemiologist	
Geneticist	
Hydrologist	Ground water hydrologist (10).
Immunologist	
Meteorologist	Air pollution meteorologist (10).
Microbiologist (9)	Bacteriologist.

Primary title *(1)*	Alternate title
	Mycologist.
	Parasitologist.
	Virologist.
Nutritionist *(11)*	
Oceanographer	Estuarine oceanographer *(10)*.
Pathologist	
Pharmacologist	Toxicologist.
Physicist	Biophysicist.
	Health physicist *(10)*.
Physiologist	
Sanitary sciences specialist *(10)*	
Zoologist	Limnologist *(10)*.

17. Nursing and Related Services:
    Nurse — Registered nurse–R.N.
    Graduate nurse.
    Professional nurse.
    Hospital nurse.
    Occupational health (industrial) nurse.
    Office nurse.
    Private duty nurse.
    Public health nurse.
    School nurse.
    Nurse anesthetist.
    Nurse midwife *(12)*.
    Obstetrical nurse.
    Pediatric nurse.
    Psychiatric nurse.
    Surgical (operating room) nurse.

    Practical nurse — Licensed practical nurse.
    Vocational nurse.
    Licensed vocational nurse.

    Nursing aide
    Orderly — Nursing assistant.
    Attendant
    Home health aide — Psychiatric (mental health) aide.
    Home aide–homemaker.
    Visiting health aide.

    Ward clerk — Floor clerk.
18. Occupational Therapy:
    Occupational therapist
    Occupational therapy assistant — Occupational therapy technician
    Occupational therapy aide
19. Orthotic and Prosthetic Technology:
    Orthotist — Orthopedic brace maker.
    Orthotic aide
    Prosthetist — Artificial limb maker.
    Prosthetic aide
    Restoration technician
20. Pharmacy:
    Pharmacist — Community pharmacist.
    Hospital pharmacist.

Primary title (*1*)	Alternate title
	Industrial pharmacist.
Pharmacy aide	Pharmacy helper.
21. Physical Therapy:	
Physical therapist	
Physical therapy assistant	Physical therapy technician.
Physical therapy aide	
22. Podiatric Medicine:	
Podiatrist	Chiropodist.
	Foot orthopedist.
	Foot roentgenologist.
	Podiatric surgeon.
	Pododermatologist.
23. Radiologic Technology:	
Radiologic technologist	
Radiologic technician	X-ray technician.
	Radiation therapy technician.
24. Secretarial and Office Services (*4*):	
Secretary	Dental secretary.
	Medical secretary.
Office assistant	Dentist's office assistant.
	Medical assistant.
	Optometrist's office assistant.
	Physician's office assistant.
25. Social Sciences (*4*):	
Anthropologist	Cultural (social) anthropologist.
	Physical anthropologist.
Economist	Health economist.
Psychologist	Clinical psychologist.
	Counseling psychologist.
	Measurement psychologist (psychometrist).
	Social psychologist.
Sociologist	Medical sociologist.
26. Social Work:	
Clinical social worker	Medical social worker.
	Psychiatric social worker.
Clinical social work assistant	
Clinical social work aide	Clinical casework aide.
27. Specialized Rehabilitation Services:	
Corrective therapist	
Corrective therapy aide	
Educational therapist	
Manual arts therapist	
Music therapist	
Recreation therapist	Therapeutic recreation specialist.
Recreation therapy aide	
Homemaking rehabilitation consultant	
28. Speech Pathology and Audiology:	
Audiologist	Hearing therapist.
Speech pathologist	Speech therapist.

Primary title (1)	*Alternate title*
29. Veterinary Medicine: Veterinarian	Laboratory (animal medicine) veterinarian. Public health veterinarian. Veterinary laboratory diagnostician. Veterinary microbiologist. Veterinary pathologist. Veterinary radiologist. Veterinary surgeon. Veterinary toxicologist.
Veterinary technician	Animal technician.
30. Vision Care and Services: Ophthalmologist (13) Optometrist Vision care technologist	Ocular care technologist. Ophthalmic technologist. Optometric technologist.
Technician: Vision care technician	Ocular care technician. Ophthalmic technician (assistant). Optometric technician (assistant).
Orthoptic technician	Orthoptist.
Optician	Dispensing optician. Ophthalmic dispenser (optical fitter). Contact lens technician. Lens grinder-polisher (14). Optical (laboratory) mechanic.
Vision care aide	Ocular care aide. Ophthalmic aide. Optometric aide. Visual training aide.
31. Vocational Rehabilitation Counseling: Vocational rehabilitation counselor	Rehabilitation counselor.
32. Miscellaneous Health Services: Assistance for physicians: Physician's associate (15)	Child health associate. Pediatric associate.
Physician's assistant	Anesthetic assistant. Orthopedic assistant.
Physician's aide	Obstetrical aide. Pediatric aide. Surgical aide.
Emergency health service: Medical emergency technician Ambulance attendant (aide) Inhalation therapy: Inhalation therapist Inhalation therapy aide Medical machine technology:	 Inhalation therapy technician.

Primary title (1)	Alternate title
Cardiopulmonary technician	
Electrocardiograph technician	
Electroencephalograph technician	
Other	Biomedical instrument technician.
Nuclear medicine:	
Nuclear medical technologist	
Nuclear medical technician	
Other health services:	
Community health aide	Dental health aide.
	Mental health aide (worker).
	School health aide.
Extracorporeal circulation specialist	
Other	

(1) The occupations listed are those which make a significant contribution to the health field and for which individuals have developed specialized competence.

(2) Includes pathology laboratory.

(3) See Natural Sciences.

(4) For some of the occupations listed, only a minority of the workers may be engaged in health related work.

(5) Includes specialists in pediatric allergy and cardiology.

(6) Includes specialists in child psychiatry.

(7) Includes specialists in diagnostic and therapeutic radiology.

(8) See Nursing and Related Services.

(9) See Clinical Laboratory Services.

(10) See Environmental Health Activities.

(11) See Dietetic and Nutritional Services.

(12) See Midwifery.

(13) See Medicine and Osteopathy.

(14) Also known as assembler, benchman, edger, or surfacer; optical technician or shopman.

(15) Baccalaureate or higher educational background.

Source: *Health Resources Statistics,* 1971. National Center for Health Statistics, U.S. Department of HEW, PHS, HSMHA (Rockville, Maryland), February 1972.

Table 2-2. Estimated Persons Employed in Selected Occupations Within Each Health Field: 1970

Health field and occupation	Workers
Total[1]	4,182,140 to 4,365,340
Administration of health services	48,000 to 49,000
Administrator, program representative, management officer	48,000 to 49,000
Anthropology and sociology	1,400 to 1,600

Health field and occupation	*Workers*
Anthropologist—cultural and physical	600
Sociologist—medical	800 to 1,000
Automatic data processing in the health field	1,500 to 2,500
Systems analyst	1,500 to 2,500
Basic sciences in the health field	51,200
Research scientist (other than physician, dentist, veterinarian)	[2]51,200
Biomedical engineering	10,700 to 10,900
Biomedical engineer	3,500 to 3,700
Biomedical engineering technician	7,200
Chiropractic and naturopathy	16,000 to 18,000
Chiropractor, naturopath, other drugless healer	[2]16,000 to 18,000
Clinical laboratory services	140,000
Clinical laboratory scientist	5,000
Clinical (medical) laboratory technologist	70,000
Clinical laboratory technician and assistant	65,000
Dentistry and allied services	240,900 to 245,900
Dentist	[3]102,900
Dental hygienist	16,000
Dental assistant	90,000 to 95,000
Dental laboratory technician	32,000
Dietetic and nutritional services	47,000
Dietitian and nutritionist	[4]30,000
Dietary technician, food service supervisor	17,000
Economic research in the health field	300 to 500
Economist—health	300 to 500
Environmental control	242,000
Environmental engineer	35,000
Scientist	25,000
Sanitarian	12,000
Technician	69,000
Aide	101,000
Food and drug protective services	21,640 to 26,640
Food technologist	20,000 to 25,000
Food and drug analyst and inspector	1,640

Health field and occupation	Workers
Health and vital statistics	[2]1,350
Health statistician	1,100
Vital record registrar	150
Demographer	100
Health education	22,000 to 23,000
Public health educator	[2]2,000 to 3,000
School health educator, coordinator	20,000
Health information and communication	10,500 to 12,600
Biological photographer	2,000
Health information specialist and service writer	[2]2,000 to 3,000
Health technical writer	6,000 to 7,000
Medical illustrator	[2]500 to 600
Library services in the health field	9,500
Medical librarian	2,200
Medical library technician and clerk	7,300
Medical records	53,000
Medical record administrator	11,000
Medical record technician	42,000
Medicine and osteopathy	323,000
Physician (M.D.)	[3]311,000
Physician (D.O.)	[3]12,000
Midwifery	5,300
Lay midwife	4,100
Nurse-midwife	1,200
Nursing and related services	1,990,000 to 1,995,000
Registered nurse	723,000
Practical nurse	400,000
Nursing aide, orderly, attendant	850,000
Home health aide	17,000 to 22,000
Occupational therapy	12,800
Occupational therapist	7,300
Occupational therapy technician, assistant	5,500
Optometry and opticianry	34,700 to 35,200

Health filed and occupation	*Workers*
Optometrist	[5] 18,400
Dispensing optician	11,000
Optometric assistant	4,500 to 5,000
Optometric technician	800
Orthotic and prosthetic technology	3,600
Orthotist and prosthetist	[2] 3,600
Pharmacy	139,300
Pharmacist	[3] 129,300
Pharmacy assistant and aide	10,000
Physical therapy	24,000
Physical therapist	15,000
Physical therapy technician, assistant	9,000
Podiatry	[3] 7,000
Podiatrist	7,000
Psychology	13,000
Psychologist—clinical, counseling, and other health	13,000
Radiologic technology	75,000 to 100,000
Radiologic (X-ray) technologist, technician, assistant	[2] 75,000 to 100,000
Secretarial and office services in the health field	275,000 to 300,000
Receptionist, secretary, assistant, aide	275,000 to 300,000
Social work	29,800
Social worker—medical and psychiatric	25,500
Social work assistant and aide	[6] 4,300
Specialized rehabilitation services	11,300
Corrective therapist	1,200
Educational therapist	[5] 500
Manual arts therapist	[5] 900
Music therapist	[2] 2,200
Therapeutic recreational specialist	6,000
Home economist in rehabilitation	[2] 500
Speech pathology and audiology	19,000
Speech pathologist and audiologist	19,000
Veterinary medicine	[3] 25,700
Veterinarian	25,700
Vocational rehabilitation counseling	13,400
Vocational rehabilitation counselor	13,400

Health field and occupation	*Workers*
Miscellaneous health services	268,250 to 373,250
Ambulance attendant	5,600
Electrocardiograph technician	9,500
Electroencephalograph technician	3,300
Inhalation therapy technician	11,000
Medical assistant	200,000 to 300,000
Ophthalmic assistant	15,000 to 20,000
Orthoptist	450
Surgical aide and other aides	23,400

[1] Each occupation is counted only once. For example, all physicians are in medicine and osteopathy.

[2] 1968 estimate repeated in absence of sufficient information on which to base revision.

[3] Estimate indicates active rather than total.

[4] 1965 estimate repeated in absence of sufficient information on which to base revision.

[5] 1969 estimate.

[6] Limited to hospital employees in 1969.

Source: *Health Resources Statistics,* 1971. National Center for Health Statistics, U.S. Dept. of HEW, PHS, HSMHA (Rockville, Maryland), February 1972.

Table 2-3.   Accrediting Agencies for Educational Programs

Educational Program	*Accrediting Agencies (Granting Approval of the Educational Program)* *
Certified Laboratory Assistant	1) Council on Medical Education or the American Medical Association (AMA) 2) American Society of Clinical Pathologists (ASCP) 3) American Society of Medical Technologists
Cytotechnology	1) Council on Medical Education (AMA) 2) Board of Schools of Medical Technology of the ASCP
Dental Hygiene	Council on Dental Education of the American Dental Association (ADA)
Dentistry	Council on Dental Education (ADA)
Dietetics	American Dietetic Association
Hospital Administration	Accrediting Commission on Graduate Education for Hospital Administration
Inhalation Therapy	1) Council on Medical Education (AMA) 2) American Association for Inhalation Therapy 3) American Society of Anesthesiologists 4) American College of Chest Physicians

Educational Program	*Accrediting Agencies* *(Granting Approval of the Educational Program)* *
Library Science (Special courses in hospital and medical library science)	1) American Library Association 2) Medical Library Association
Medical Illustration	Council on Education of the Association of Medical Illustrators
Medical Records	1) Council on Medical Education (AMA) 2) Committee on Education and Registration
Medical Technology	1) Council on Medical Education (AMA) 2) Board of Schools of Medical Technology (ASCP) 3) American Society of Medical Technologists
Medical Schools	1) Council on Medical Education (AMA) 2) Association of American Medical Colleges
Nurse Anesthesia	American Association of Nurse Anesthetists
Practical Nursing	Listed and approved by state government agencies
Professional Nursing	a) Listed and approved by state government agencies b) The National League for Nursing also accredits nursing schools
Occupational Therapy	1) Council on Medical Education (AMA) 2) American Occupational Therapy Association
Occupational Therapy Assistants	American Occupational Therapy Association
Operating Room Technicians	Association of Operating Room Nurses
Osteopathy	American Osteopathic Association
Pharmacy	American Council on Pharmaceutical Education
Physical Therapy	1) Council on Medical Education (AMA) 2) American Physical Therapy Association
Podiatry	Council on Podiatry Education, American Podiatry Association
Public Health	American Public Health Association
Radiation Therapy Technology and Radiologic Technology	1) Council on Medical Education (AMA) 2) American College of Radiology 3) American Society of Radiologic Technologists
Social Work	Council on Social Work Education
Speech Pathology and Audiology	American Speech and Hearing Association

*Numbered agencies mean there is a joint accreditation program.

Source: 1971 Guide Issue, *Hospitals, JAHA.* This lists names and addresses of health organizations.

Table 2-4.   Calendar for Health Career Education*

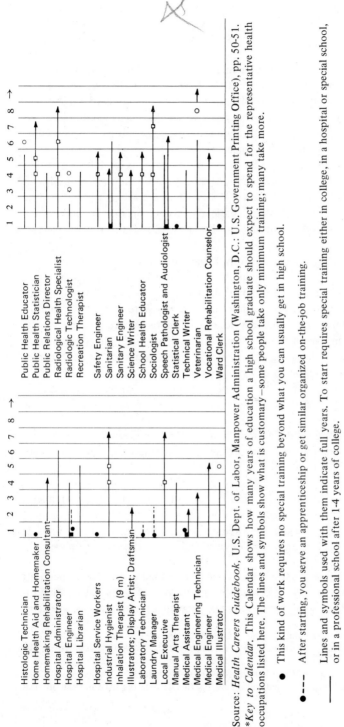

Histologic Technician
Home Health Aid and Homemaker
Homemaking Rehabilitation Consultant
Hospital Administrator
Hospital Engineer
Hospital Librarian

Hospital Service Workers
Industrial Hygienist
Inhalation Therapist (9 m)
Illustrators; Display Artist; Draftsman
Laboratory Technician
Laundry Manager
Local Executive
Manual Arts Therapist
Medical Assistant
Medical Engineering Technician
Medical Engineer
Medical Illustrator

Public Health Educator
Public Health Statistician
Public Relations Director
Radiological Health Specialist
Radiologic Technologist
Recreation Therapist

Safety Engineer
Sanitarian
Sanitary Engineer
Science Writer
School Health Educator
Sociologist
Speech Pathologist and Audiologist
Statistical Clerk
Technical Writer
Veterinarian
Vocational Rehabilitation Counselor
Ward Clerk

Source: *Health Careers Guidebook*, U.S. Dept. of Labor, Manpower Administration (Washington, D.C.: U.S. Government Printing Office), pp. 50-51.
Key to Calendar. This Calendar shows how many years of education a high school graduate should expect to spend for the representative health occupations listed here. The lines and symbols show what is customary—some people take only minimum training; many take more.

●   This kind of work requires no special training beyond what you can usually get in high school.

●‒‒‒   After starting, you serve an apprenticeship or get similar organized on-the-job training.

| Lines and symbols used with them indicate full years. To start requires special training either in college, in a hospital or special school, or in a professional school after 1-4 years of college.

⌐   Special training is required, but you have a choice, each type of training taking a different number of years.

□   First symbol means you can get beginner's job after college, but will usually need more study, as well as experience, for advancement. Graduate training ordinarily goes to or beyond master's or doctor's degree.

↑   Your planning should look beyond minimum requirements; continuing study, after entering professional practice, is important to further advancement.

○   Though the line shows the minimum to qualify, more preprofessional years in college often lengthen the total training time.

(9m)   Special course or on-the-job training is shown in number of months.

2. PHYSICIANS

Physician (M.D.) Education

The educational requirements for the training of physicians was largely cast in its present mold as a result of the *Flexner Report*[5] in 1910, in which Abraham Flexner criticized many of the medical schools of his day. The American Medical Association then undertook to accredit medical schools, classifying them as "A," "B," or "C," depending on their performance. Since 1938, only "A" rated medical schools have existed.

Admission to medical school requires three years of college, although four years and a B.A. degree are preponderant. Also required are a number of *pre-medical* college courses. These vary somewhat according to the medical school, but usually include biology, basic chemistry, organic chemistry, and physics. The *Medical College Admissions Test* (MCAT) is also used to evaluate the applicant's potential.

Traditionally, medical schools[6] have had four-year programs, typically divided into two years of pre-clinical or basic science courses and two years of clinical courses and practical training, the latter mostly in teaching hospitals.

A decade ago, medical school curriculums were very similar in most schools. In the interval there has developed considerable variation among the schools, including an overall trend toward increased elective time. Many schools have developed accelerated programs whereby requirements for the M.D. degree may be completed in 36 months or less.

There are 114 medical schools. Of these, six provide two years of basic medical sciences, after which students may transfer to advanced standing in a four-year school.

Medical schools are accredited by the *Liaison Committee on Medical Education,* a joint committee of the Association of American Medical Colleges and the AMA.

National Boards. The National Board examinations are standard, national examinations developed and administered by the National Board of Medical Examiners. They are given in three parts which are generally taken during the second and the final medical schools years and during the internship year.

Internship and Residency Training (Graduate Medical Education). After medical school, nearly all physicians enter a year of hospital-based internship. There are two general types: *straight,* providing training in one specialty

---

[5]Flexner, Abraham, *Medical Education in the United States and Canada, A Report to the Carnegie Foundation for the Advancement of Teaching,* (New York: The Carnegie Foundation, 1910).

[6]Medical schools are either state or privately owned and, almost always, part of a university. They are represented nationally by the Association of American Medical Colleges (AAMC).

such as Internal Medicine or Surgery; and *rotating,* including more than two specialty areas.

Selection of an internship is processed by the National Intern Matching Program, which uses a computer program to match applicant and hospital preferences.

In the past, all internship programs have been approved by the A. M.A.'s Council on Medical Education. By 1975, all internships will be coordinated with residency programs and will be designated as *categorical* (straight) and *flexible.* All will be approved by the appropriate specialty bodies and the new Liaison Committee on Graduate Medical Education.

✕ **Specialization.** After internship, most physicians take further specialty training in a residency program of two to five years' duration depending on the field. These programs are approved by specialty residency review committees and the Liaison Committee on Graduate Medical Education.[7] Training during this period may also include *fellowships* (usually for research or special studies). Also, most male physicians have been required to serve for two years or more in the armed services (*the doctor draft*) or in the Public Health Service (See Table 2-5).

After specialty training, a physician who wishes to be certified will apply to the appropriate *specialty board.*[8] The requirements for certification by a specialty board include completion of an approved internship and residency program,[9] written and oral examination, and varying years of practice. Completing all these requirements makes a physician *board certified* or a *diplomate* of that board.

✕ **Specialty Boards.** Specialties and their specialty boards are recognized and approved by the American Board of Medical Specialties in conjunction with the AMA Council on Medical Education.

There are 20 *primary* boards:

Anesthesiology
Colon and Rectal Surgery (Proctology)
Dermatology
Family Practice
Internal Medicine
Neurological Surgery (Neuro-Surgery)
Obstetrics-Gynecology

---

[7]This committee includes representatives from the American Board of Medical Specialties, American Hospital Association, American Medical Association, American Association of Medical Colleges and the Council of Medical Specialty Societies.

[8]A physician need not, however, be certified by a specialty board in order to practice a specialty.

Table 2-5. Modal Physician's Progress*

Educational Institution	Usual Number of Years	Usual Requirements	Modal Age at Graduation
High School	12		17-18 years
College	4	Pre-Medical Courses MCAT	21-22
Medical School	4	2 Pre-Clinical Years 2 Clinical Years	25-26
Internship	1	Completion of National Board Exams, State Licensure	26-27
Residency	2-5+	May also include fellowship	28-32+
Military Service	2	May include internship and/or residency or come prior to residency	30-34+
Specialty Requirements → Specialty Practice		Examinations, Experience and Others	
General Practice	—		

Graduate of Foreign Medical Schools

ECFMG Exam

and other careers (Research, Teaching, Administrative, etc.)

*See American Medical Association, *Directory of Approved Internships and Residencies, 1971-1972.* The Association, Chicago, Illinois, p. 9.

Ophthalmology
Orthopedic Surgery
Otolaryngology
Pathology
Pediatrics
Physical Medicine and Rehabilitation
Plastic Surgery
Preventive Medicine[10]
Psychiatry and Neurology
Radiology
Surgery (General Surgery)
Thoracic Surgery
Urology

In addition to these 20 boards, there are 5 *subsidiary* (subspecialty) boards:

Cardiovascular Disease (Internal Medicine)
Child Psychiatry (Psychiatry and Neurology)
Gastroenterology (Internal Medicine)
Pediatric Cardiology (Pediatrics)
Pulmonary Disease (Internal Medicine)

There are also two *conjoint boards* based on cooperation of two or more primary boards:

1) *Nuclear Medicine,* a conjoint board of Internal Medicine, Pathology and Radiology.
2) *Allergy and Immunology,* a conjoint board of Internal Medicine and Pediatrics.

Additional subspecialties are recognized, such as endocrinology and metabolism, hematology, infectious disease, nephrology (kidney disease) and rheumatology (subspecialties of Internal Medicine), pediatric allergy, forensic pathology, and others. An emerging specialty, with newly developed residency programs, is Emergency Medicine.

There are also general practice residency programs, many of which have been modified to meet the requirements of the new specialty board of Family Practice.

Licensure. Medical licensure is on a state-by-state basis. If a physician is licensed in one state, it does not allow him to practice medicine in another

---

[10]Certifies specialists in Public Health, Aerospace Medicine, Occupational Medicine or General Preventive Medicine.

state without obtaining its license. (Special temporary state licenses are granted to resident physicians working in hospitals.)

In all states, the requirements, which are set forth in Medical Practice Acts, include passing an examination. Traditionally, these have been developed and administered by state boards. In many states, certification by the National Board of Medical Examiners is accepted in lieu of state examinations.

In recent years, there has been wide acceptance by the states of the Federation Licensing Examination (FLEX),[11] developed by the Federation of Licensing Boards.

Many states recognize, in lieu of examination, licenses granted by certain other states (reciprocity).

Foreign Medical Graduates. Graduates of foreign medical schools (except Canadian) who wish to take an approved U.S. internship or residency must pass an examination prepared by the Educational Council for Foreign Medical Graduates (ECFMG).[12]

Osteopathic Physicians (D.O.)

Physicians (M.D.) and *Osteopathic Physicians (D.O.)* are often grouped together because their education and mode of practice are quite similar. Until recently, *osteopathy* and *medicine* have constituted separate professions with separate education and hospitals. Recently there has been more interchange between the two.

Osteopathy originated as a reform movement in American medicine, originally propounded in 1874 by Dr. Andrew Taylor Still. Today there are seven colleges of osteopathy accredited by the American Osteopathic Association, whose graduates receive the degree of Doctor of Osteopathy (D.O.).

The content of osteopathic education is the same as that in M.D. medical schools except that osteopaths have additional class hours devoted to osteopathic manipulation.

Over time, differences in approaches to treatment between medicine and osteopathy have narrowed to the point where, in California, these two professions have completely merged.

Osteopathy has been defined (1956) as "a system of medical practice based on the theory that disease is due chiefly to mechanical derangement in tissues, placing emphasis on restoration of structural integrity by manipulation of the parts. The uses of medicines, surgery, proper diet, psychotherapy, and other measures are included in osteopathy."

---

[11] John P. Hubbard, "Evaluation, Certification and Licensure in Medicine," *JAMA* 225, 4 (July 23, 1973): 401.

[12] The Council is sponsored by the American Hospital Association, the American Medical Association, the Association of American Medical Colleges, the Association for Hospital and Medical Education and the Federation of State Medical Boards.

In 1963, about half of the 12,000 practicing osteopaths were located in Michigan, Missouri, Ohio, Pennsylvania, and Texas (excluding California, where M.D.'s and D.O.'s have merged). In recent years, over 70 percent of the students entering osteopathic colleges have a bachelor's degree. One year of internship after the D.O. degree is customary, and beyond that there is further training leading to membership in one of twelve osteopathic specialty boards. While most M.D.'s specialize, most D.O.'s practice family medicine. Licensure is required for practice. Nearly all states grant osteopathic physicians the same practice privileges as medical physicians, although a few states restrict osteopathic use of drugs and surgery.

Table 2-6 shows the number of medical and osteopathic physicians in various specialties.

The word "medicine" is used in three ways. One is to refer to all activities of physicians (as in "the practice of medicine"). The second use is in distinction to "surgery" (as in "internal medicine"). The third use is to distinguish medicine from osteopathy.

Table 2-6. Type of Practice and Primary Specialty of Active Federal and Non-Federal Physicians: 1967 and 1970

Primary specialty	Total active[1]	*M.D.'s (Dec. 31, 1970)* Patient care				D.O.'s (Dec. 31, 1967)
		Office-based practice[2]	Hospital-based practice Training programs	Full-time physician staff	Other professional activity[3]	
Total	310,845	192,439	51,228	34,868	32,310	[4]11,381
General practice[5]	77,363	54,914	10,400	5,946	6,103	[6]8,651
Specialty practice	233,482	137,525	40,828	28,922	26,207	1,416
Medical specialties	77,214	44,428	14,139	8,646	10,001	354
Allergy	1,719	1,395	61	66	197	2
Cardiovascular diseases	6,476	3,905	568	711	1,292	2
Dermatology	4,003	2,967	556	237	253	20
Gastroenterology	2,010	1,117	221	212	460	–
Internal medicine	41,872	23,284	8,965	4,511	5,112	266
Pediatrics[7]	18,819	10,958	3,567	2,186	2,108	64
Pulmonary diseases	2,315	812	201	723	579	–
Surgical specialties	96,902	66,650	16,880	8,664	4,708	841
Anesthesiology	10,860	7,379	1,408	1,326	747	180
Colon and rectal surgery	667	605	22	21	19	43

Primary specialty	Total active[1]	M.D.'s (Dec. 31, 1970)				D.O.'s (Dec. 31, 1967)
		Patient care			Other professional activity[3]	
			Hospital-based practice			
		Office-based practice[2]	Training programs	Full-time physician staff		
General surgery	29,761	18,229	7,142	2,985	1,405	273
Neurological surgery	2,578	1,671	520	235	152	5
Obstetrics and gynecology	18,876	13,910	2,519	1,458	989	80
Ophthalmology	9,927	7,662	1,334	517	414	133
Orthopedic surgery	9,620	6,569	1,834	895	322	73
Otolaryngology	5,409	3,949	814	419	227	23
Plastic surgery	1,600	1,171	256	113	60	1
Thoracic surgery	1,809	1,215	199	240	155	5
Urology	5,795	4,290	832	455	218	25
Psychiatry and neurology	26,310	12,595	4,289	5,465	3,961	31
Child psychiatry	2,090	1,071	315	319	385	–
Neurology	3,074	1,212	696	478	688	3
Psychiatry	21,146	10,312	3,278	4,668	2,888	28
Other specialties	33,056	13,852	5,520	6,147	7,537	190
Aerospace medicine	1,188	415	74	241	458	–
General preventive medicine	804	183	44	55	522	–
Occupational medicine	2,713	1,920	16	79	698	3
Pathology[8]	10,483	3,128	2,278	2,573	2,504	46
Physical medicine and rehabilitation	1,479	549	236	519	175	9
Public health	3,029	526	96	184	2,223	–
Radiology[9]	13,360	7,131	2,776	2,496	957	132

[1] Excludes 3,204 M.D.'s with addresses unknown, and 358 unclassified M.D.'s.

[2] Previously called solo, partnership, group, or other practice.

[3] Includes medical teaching, administration, research, and other.

[4] Includes 1,314 D.O.'s (775 in training programs, 181 in full-time hospital staff positions, 186 in other professional activities, and 172 federal D.O.'s) for whom data are not available on specialties.

[5] Includes no specialty reported and other specialties not listed.

[6] Includes 827 with practice limited to manipulative therapy.

[7] Includes pediatric allergy and pediatric cardiology.

[8] Includes forensic pathology.

[9] Includes diagnostic roentgenology and therapeutic radiology.

Source: *Health Resource Statistics, 1971.* National Center for Health Statistics, USDHEW, PHS, HSMHA (Rockville, Maryland), February 1972.

From: AMA Center for Health Services Research and Development: *Distribution of Physicians in the United States, 1970. Regional, State, County, Metropolitan Areas.* J.N. Haug, G.A. Roback and B.C. Martin, Chicago, American Medical Association, 1971. AOA Membership and Statistics Department: *A Statistical Study of the Osteopathic Profession,* December 31, 1967, Chicago, American Osteopathic Association, June 1968.

References

American Medical Association, *Directory of Approved Internships and Residencies* (Chicago: The Association, Yearly).

Association of American Medical Colleges, *Medical School Admissions Requirements* (Washington, D.C.: The Association, Yearly).

Advisory Board for Medical Specialists, Inc., *The Directory of Medical Specialists,* Fifteenth Edition (Chicago: Marquis-Who's Who, 1972-1973).

"Medical Education in the United States," *Journal of the American Medical Association,* November, Yearly.

Rosemary Stevens, *American Medicine and the Public Interest* (New Haven: Yale University Press, 1971). A study of the evolution of medical specialization in the United States.

3. DENTISTS

A minimum of two years of college is required for admission to dental school. About 50 percent of dental students have a bachelor's degree, and this percentage is increasing. Most dental schools require four academic years to obtain the D.M.D. (Doctor of Dental Medicine) or D.D.S. (Doctor of Dental Surgery) degree, although some now have a three calendar year program. For all practical purposes, there is no difference in the D.M.D. and D.D.S. degrees. Dentists and Physicians are both Doctors, so it is inappropriate to say "Dentists and Doctors."

To be admitted to dental school it is necessary to take the Dental Aptitude Test (DAT) prepared by the Division of Educational Measurements of the American Dental Association (ADA). In the first two years (basic science years) of dental school, in some universities, the dental students take the same courses as the medical students, with the addition of oral anatomy, oral pathology, and other pre-clinical dental science courses. The third and fourth years are usually the clinical years, when students treat patients under faculty supervision in the school's clinics or community facilities. Now some schools are blending the basic sciences and clinical years. Dental internships and residencies are not required for general practice, but are required for board certification in a dental specialty. The eight recognized dental specialties are:

1. *Endodontics* (root treatment).
2. *Oral Pathology* (the study of diseased oral tissues).
3. *Oral Surgery*
4. *Orthodontics* (straightening of the teeth).
5. *Pedodontics* (children's dentistry).
6. *Periodontology* or *Periodontics* (treatment of the gums, bone, and other tissues surrounding the teeth).
7. *Prosthodontics* (replacing missing teeth).
8. *Public Health Dentistry*

In addition to the dental degree, all states and the District of Columbia require a written and practical examination for licensure. A certificate from the National Board of Dental Examiners is accepted in place of the written exam in all states except Delaware and Arizona.[13] Regional Dental Examining Boards have been established and successful completion of those examinations is accepted as satisfying the practical examination requirement for several specified states.

Canadian dental education is accepted in most states, but graduates from other foreign dental schools must take additional training in a U.S. Dental School before being examined for licensure. The Science Achievement Examination for Dentistry allows up to 2 years advance placement in a U.S. Dental School. The foreign graduate must take the last two clinical years in a U.S. Dental School.

About 90 percent of active dentists are in private practice and most are in general practice, although specialization is increasing. Other careers include research, teaching, and administration. There is a growing interest in allied dental occupations including:

1. *Dental Hygienist*—requires two years of formal education and training as well as state licensure.
2. *Dental Assistant*—assists the dentist in patient care (no educational requirements although there are many dental assistant training programs of one or more years' duration. National examination and certification is possible).
3. *Dental Laboratory Technicians*—(sometimes called Denturists in Canada) who perform certain mechanical and technical procedures involved in the fabrication of artificial teeth and dentures.

Emerging programs train *Dental Therapists, Expanded Duty Auxiliaries,* or *Expanded Duty Dental Assistants* (EDDAs). This development is similar in concept to Physician's Assistants. These new personnel undertake a wider range of tasks than dental hygienists, but a smaller range than dentists. Dental schools are now providing courses for dentists in Dental Auxiliary Utilization (DAU) and Training in Expanded Auxiliary Management (TEAM).

4. NURSES

The following is a brief description of nursing, particularly nursing education, which is designed to provide a basic background for the many current issues and changes in the field, and its relation to other health professions.

---

[13] *Manpower Supply and Educational Statistics for Dentists and Dental Auxiliaries,* U.S. Dept. of HEW, Public Health Service, Bethesda, Md. (April 1972), p. 1.

Professional Nurses

Professional nurses are generally known in the United States as registered nurses (RNs). (In the past the terms *graduate* and *trained nurse* have also been used.)

Education. There are three basic types of educational programs which prepare registered nurses: diploma, baccalaureate, and associate degree.

Diploma programs. These are typically three-year programs in hospital-based schools of nursing. These schools had their origin in the training schools for nursing which began to be established in the 1870s and which were originally based on the nursing education principles newly established in London by Florence Nightingale.[14]

Until recently, the great majority of nursing graduates came from diploma schools. With the increasing development of college programs, the percentage of diploma graduates has declined and the total number of such programs is diminishing.[15]

Baccalaureate programs. These are four-or five-year college or university-based programs which lead to the Bachelor of Science degree. Clinical experience is obtained in university or affiliated teaching hospitals.

The first school established within a university was at the University of Minnesota (1910). Such schools began to come to prominence in the 1930s and have steadily expanded in numbers; in 1969-70 they graduated 21 percent of new nurses.

Associate degree programs. These are two-year programs, usually based in junior and community colleges, leading to an Associate in Arts degree. Practical experience is obtained in affiliated hospitals. Such programs were first established in 1952[16] and have rapidly increased, graduating 27 percent of new nurses in 1969-70.

Nursing educational programs are approved by state agencies, such as the state education department or nursing board. In addition, a voluntary

---

[14]The first three of these schools were the Bellevue Training School for Nurses, the Connecticut Training School (New Haven) and Massachusetts General Hospital Training School (all established in 1873).

Significant for the future development of nursing education in the United States was the fact that most of these schools were developed as integral parts of hospitals and became closely associated with the provision of hospital nursing services in an essentially apprentice system.

[15]Contributing to the decline in the hospital programs has been the increased costs associated with improved curriculums and decreased emphasis on meeting hospital service needs.

[16]By seven colleges in cooperation with the Cooperative Research Project in Junior and Community College Education, Teachers College, Columbia University.

accreditation program is carried out by the National League for Nursing and most schools and programs are so accredited.

Licensure. The first licensure acts for nurses were passed in 1903, and by 1923 all states and the District of Columbia had such laws. These statutes, usually called *nursing practice acts* are administered by nursing boards.[17]

In a few states, licensure is not mandatory for the practice of nursing; their licensure laws merely prohibiting unlicensed persons from using the title "registered nurse;" i.e., these laws are voluntary, protecting the title, but not regulating nursing practice. Licensure examinations, required in all states, are administered by the nursing boards, from an examination pool maintained by the National League of Nursing.

Advanced Training and Specialization. There are many *master's degree* programs which have been developed for the advanced training of nurses in nursing education, administration, and clinical specialties.[18]

The clinical specialty programs include public health (community health), medical-surgical nursing, maternal and child health, mental health, rehabilitation, and cardiovascular nursing.

A number of *doctoral degree* programs in nursing have been established since the mid-1940s. This level of education is being encouraged by many nursing educators for nurses pursuing teaching and research careers in collegiate programs.

"Nurse-clinicians, clinical nursing specialists." The increasing popularity of educational programs in the clinical specialties is a manifestation of a trend toward making available opportunities for professional advancement for nurses by increasing clinical skills as opposed to the traditional routes of teaching or administration.[19] Other examples of the development of special clinical skills are the hospital in-service training programs for nurses in intensive care and coronary care units; and the *nurse practitioner* programs which have been developed in ambulatory care settings (see Chapter 6).

A related development has been the trend toward relieving nurses of non-nursing administrative and clerical tasks in order that more of their energy can be devoted to patient care. One manifestation of this trend has been the establishment of *ward manager,* (unit manager) positions in many hospitals.

---

[17]Variously named Board of Nursing, Board of Nursing Examiners, Board of Nursing Education and Nurse Registration, etc.

[18]Advanced education for professional nurses had its origins in programs established at Teachers College, Columbia University: a course for those who would be teaching in nursing schools (1900) and courses in public health nursing (1910).

[19]For example, the usual route for advancement in hospital nursing has been from staff nurse to head nurse, nursing supervisor, assistant director, and, ultimately, director of nurses.

Two older types of nurse specialists are particularly noteworthy: *nurse midwives* and *nurse anesthetists*.

Nurse Anesthetists. Nurse anesthetists have been employed in hospital surgical units since before 1900 and the first school for the formal training of nurses in the administration of anesthesia was established at Lakeside Hospital in Cleveland about 1910. Programs now are generally of 18-months' duration and lead to certification.

Nurse Midwives. [20] Nurse midwives are registered nurses with special training in prenatal and postpartum care and the management of normal labor and delivery.

The first U.S. training school was established in New York City in 1932. Nurse midwives trained in Britain had been practicing with the Frontier Nursing Service in Kentucky since 1927, and a School of Midwifery was established there in 1939.

Programs, leading to certification, are from 8-24 months, the latter leading to a master's degree.

Practical Nurses

Practical nurses are recognized in all states as *licensed* practical nurses (LPN) or as licensed *vocational* nurses (LVN) (California and Texas).

The first educational programs in practical nursing were established under provisions of the Vocational Education Act of 1917 (Smith-Hughes Act). They are based in vocational and technical schools, hospitals and community colleges and are generally of eight to fifteen months' duration.

The licensing agency in most states is the state nursing board; there is a separate board of practical nursing examiners in several states. In about half the states, the law is compulsory, regulating practice; in the others, it is voluntary, protecting the title. [21]

Nursing Aides (Nursing Assistants)

Nursing aides are important personnel in hospitals and nursing homes. They perform many tasks related to personal care of patients. Educational requirements are those specified by the hiring institution, usually some years of high school. Training is on the job with scope, duration and formality varying greatly among institutions.

---

[20] Lay midwives, often called "granny midwives," have for many years practiced among poor populations, especially in the rural south. They are licensed in many states, although in many instances no new licenses are being issued.

[21] The term "waivered" practical nurse refers to those who, in certain states, have been licensed on the basis of previous practice, without the educational requirements.

Associations

American Nurses' Association (ANA).   This is the professional association for registered nurses and is particularly concerned with nursing practice and the nursing profession.

National League for Nursing (NLN).   This association includes registered and practical nurses, nursing aides, and other (non-nursing) persons interested in nursing. It is particularly concerned with the improvement of organized nursing services and educational programs.

American College of Nurse Midwives.   This is the professional association for nurse midwives. Its activities include the accreditation of training programs and the certification of their graduates.

American Association of Nurse Anesthetists.   This is the professional association for nurse anesthetists. The requirements for membership include a qualifying examination.

The National Federation of Licensed Practical Nurses is the professional association for practical nurses.

References

Mary M. Roberts, *American Nursing—History and Interpretation* (New York: The Macmillan Company, 1954).

Facts About Nursing: A Statistical Summary (New York: The American Nurses Association). Annually or Biannually.

Nursing and Nursing Education in the United States, Report of the Committee for the Study of Nursing Education and Report of a Survey by Josephine Goldmark (New York: The Macmillan Company, 1923).

Esther Lucille Brown, *Nursing for the Future* (New York: Russell Sage Foundation, 1948).

National Commission for the Study of Nursing and Nursing Education, *An Abstract for Action* (New York: McGraw-Hill Company, 1970).

5. A SAMPLING OF OTHER
HEALTH PROFESSIONS

Herein are a few short descriptions of a sampling of health occupations chosen to show the range and variation that exists. The number of different health occupations is steadily growing. Space does not permit inclusion of all of them.

Administration (Health Administration, Hospital Administration, Health Management, etc.)

Educational programs in health services administration are located in medical schools, schools of public health, business schools, and schools of government or public administration. Courses and degrees are provided at the baccalaureate, master, and doctorate levels. The Association of University Programs in Health Administration (AUPHA) is a voluntary organization which represents most of these programs.

Dieticians and Nutritionists

Dieticians specialize in feeding people, and their profession is largely hospital based. They can specialize in teaching, research, administration, and therapy (planning special menus and diets). The nutritionist is, in practice, an educator who often works in a public health setting. Both professions require a college education. Master and doctorate degrees are available. Dieticians ordinarily take a one-year internship, and post-college education is recommended for nutritionists. The American Dietetic Association (ADA) serves as the professional association for both groups. The dietician brings knowledge of, and skills in, nutrition and/or management to the feeding of individuals and groups. The nutritionist is concerned with carrying out nutritional programs for the promotion of health and prevention of disease, consults with other professionals, and provides education for both health professionals and the public.

Medical Record Librarians

This is primarily a hospital occupation. There are three routes to this career: (a) by experience without formal education, (b) by a twelve-month hospital certificate school which admits students with a minimum of two years of study in college, and (c) by four-year college programs which award a bachelor's degree of medical record administration or medical record science. Graduates of the four-year program are eligible to take the examination to qualify as a registered record librarian (RRL).

Medical Record Technicians

This requires from nine to twelve months after high school.

Medical Technology and Related Services

Medical Technologist. A registered medical technologist requires three years of college and one year in one of about 800 approved training schools. Afterwards, passing the examination confers the title M.T. (ASCP). This ASCP stands for the American Society for Clinical Pathologists, which helps administer the exam.

Cytotechnologist. Two years of college, six months in an approved school, and six months' experience in an acceptable laboratory are required. After this, passing the certifying exam allows one to use the designation C.T. (ASCP).

Blood Bank Technologists. These are registered medical technologists who have had an additional year's training in a blood bank school approved by the American Association of Blood Banks. The examination confers the title M.T. (ASCP) B.B.

Histologic Technicians. These require a year of supervised training in a clinical pathology laboratory, beyond high school. Examination confers certification as H.T. (ASCP).

Nuclear Medical Technology. For people with an M.T. (ASCP) or a B.S. degree in biologic or chemical sciences, plus a year's training.

Certified Laboratory Assistants. These work under the supervision of medical technologists and pathologists. It requires one year of hospital training beyond high school, and passing an examination confers the letters CLA.

Electrocardiograph (ECG or EKG) Technicians and *Electroencephalograph (EEG) Technicians.* These are trained on the job and usually require a high school education.

Occupational Therapy

Occupational therapy requires four years of college leading to a bachelor of science in occupational therapy. About thirty colleges and universities are approved for these programs. In addition, nine to ten months of clinical training is required. There is also an optional additional eighteen months of academic and clinical training for advanced standing, and some master's degree programs. Passing the national registration exam confers the degree O.T.R. *Occupational Therapy Assistants* require high school graduation plus a training program. Orthopedic and Prosthetic Appliance Makers make and fit artificial limbs. The *prosthetist* makes and fits artificial limbs and the *orthotist* makes and fits orthopedic braces, both working from a physician's prescription.

Ophthalmology

Opthalmology is a specialty in medicine. An *optician* dispenses eyeglasses prescribed by a physician. He fits and grinds glasses and contact lenses. Grinding is also done by optical wholesalers and by *optical technicians.* There are several schools of optical technology. Opticians are high school graduates who have had four to five years' apprenticeship. A few states license these two occupations. An *optometrist* has the degree Doctor of Optometry (O.D.) and is licensed to examine eyes for vision problems, disease, and other abnormalities. He prescribes and fits glasses. The American Optometric Association estimates that optometrists perform 75 percent of all eye examinations. Training requires two years of college and three to four years in a college of optometry. All states license optometrists, which requires an examination. An *orthoptist* helps people with crossed eyes, using instruction and exercises, and works under the guidance of an ophthalmologist. A college degree is required, plus a year in school or training. The American Orthoptic Council gives an examination and certification.

Pharmacy

Pharmacy is an applied physical science: the practice of preparing, preserving, and dispensing drugs and medicines. For many pharmacists it combines a professional and business career. About 80 percent of all pharmacists are in retail or community pharmacy. Some of these drug stores limit themselves to health products, while others sell a wide range of products. About 10 percent of pharmacists work in hospital-based pharmacies. The remainder works in industry, government, or teaching.

Pharmacy requires five years of education after high school for a B.S. in Pharmacy. Prior to 1960, four years were required. Of the current five years, the first two are pre-professional and the last three are professional. Transfer students are accepted after the first (one-four) and second (two-three) years from junior colleges or liberal arts schools. The three professional years include the study of pharmaceutical chemistry, pharmacognosy (the study of natural drugs from plants and animals), pharmacology (the action of drugs in the body), toxicology (the effects of poisons on the body, and antidotes), pharmacy administration, and clinical pharmacy. There are 73 pharmacy schools in the U.S. accredited by the American Council of Pharmaceutical Education. Master and doctorate degrees of pharmacy are also awarded. Licensure ordinarily requires a degree from an accredited school; an apprenticeship or internship of six months to one year under the supervision of a licensed pharmacist; and passage of the state board examination.

Physical Therapy

Physical Therapy qualifications can be obtained in three ways: (a) a four-year bachelor's degree program, (b) a twelve-month certificate course for people with a bachelor's degree, and (c) master's degree training. Physical Therapists are licensed.

Podiatry

Podiatrists or *Chiropodists* (these terms are synonymous) diagnose and treat diseases and deformities of the feet. There are five accredited schools of podiatry requiring two years of college before admission, and four years before receiving the DSC (Doctor of Surgical Chiropody) or Pod.D. (Doctor of Podiatry) degree. Internship is optional and not required for state licensure, although examination is. All states license podiatrists.

Public Health

Public Health includes a variety of specialized professional careers. Schools of public health are university-based and provide graduate education to a wide range of health personnel on the delivery of health services to large populations (in contrast to providing care to individual patients). Some major areas of education and research include:

Environmental Health (air pollution control, accident prevention, occupational medicine, industrial safety, control of radiological hazards, sewage and solid waste disposal, sanitation engineering, provision of clean water supplies, and fluoridation)
Population Studies (family planning, population control)
Demography (the study of population size, distribution, and characteristics)
Biostatistics (the application of statistics to health problems)
Nutrition (the relationship between food use and production and health)
Infectious Diseases and Tropical Public Health
Epidemiology (the study of the impact of disease on populations)
Maternal and Child Health
Public Health Nursing
Public Health Dentistry
Health Services Administration (medical care administration)

Radiology

Radiologic Technologists (also called *X-Ray Technicians*) assist the radiologist. Various forms of training are possible, including a 24-month program in an approved hospital-based school. Some of these programs extend over a four-year period and entitle the graduate to the degree of Bachelor of Science in X-Ray Technology. The hospital schools usually charge no tuition and have two to six students, on average.

Social Work

Professional social workers have two years of graduate education leading to the Master of Social Work (MSW) degree in an accredited school of social work. The curriculum combines classroom instruction and field experience covering social welfare policy and services, human behavior and social environment and social work practice. Areas of concentration include service to individuals (social case work) groups (social group work) and communities (community organization), administration, research, and social policy. Social workers practice both inside the health field and in other areas. Major practice settings include health, mental health, child welfare, family services, aging, juvenile, and adult justice, community service and planning.

There are also accredited four-year bachelor's degree programs whose graduates are usually called social work assistants or aides. *Neighborhood Aides* have a high school education or less. A major qualification is familiarity with the living conditions and values of the population being served and, they often function as liasion personnel between clients and social work staff.

Veterinary Medicine (care of animals)

Veterinarians receive the D.V.M. degree. Veterinarians are largely in private practice, often combining practice in their office with practice in an animal hospital. They take care of pets and other animals, such as race horses and breeding stock, which can be very valuable to their owners, who insist on excellent care to protect their investments. The work of veterinarians affects human health because veterinarians are involved in research on animals which has application to human medicine. There are diseases which are transmitted from animals to man, and the health of cattle, sheep, and other animals is important because these animals are sources of human food.

Other Practitioners or
Sectarian Practitioners

The American Medical Association refers to such practitioners as "cultists" and "quacks" because it is believed they do not accept the principles of modern scientific medicine. They have little or no contact with the "regular" medical occupations. According to the AMA, it is unethical for physicians to have any dealing with these practitioners. Needless to say, these practitioners view their roles and skills differently.

Chiropractics assume most illness can be cured by external physical manipulation of the spine. They are licensed in most states. Chiropractors are divided into the "straights" and the "mixers." The former use only spine manipulation; the mixers receive training in the basic sciences and combine manipulation with other treatment modalities.

Naprapaths rely on water baths and steam for therapy.

Naturopaths rely on special foods and diets.

Folk Medicine refers to home remedies based on cultural tradition, rather than on scientific evidence; e.g., the experssion "an apple a day keeps the doctor away," or the practice of always wearing a copper bracelet to stay healthy.

Faith Healers use the power of religious faith to cure illness.[22] For example, *Christian Science* does not accept the idea that medicine can cure illness;

---

[22]The Indian Health Service has encouraged some use of Navaho native faith healers as intermediaries between the Navaho Indians and modern medicine, in order to maintain Navaho tribal customs and the psychological benefits of their healing ceremonies.

only the Deity can. There are Christian Science Practitioners and Nurses who provide spiritual help, advice, and physical assistance to the ill.

Reference
Job Descriptions and Organizational Analysis for Hospitals and Related Health Services, Revised Edition (Washington, D.C.: U.S. Government Printing Office, 1971).

Chapter Three

Paying for Care

1. INTRODUCTION

There are several basic ways that health services are paid for and provided. They each have different characteristics and problems associated with them.

I. Direct, Out-of-Pocket Payment. Here the individual patient comes to an agreement (contracts) directly with the provider (doctor, hospital, etc.). Those patients who cannot pay all their bill receive care for free or less than the usual price as a form of *charity*. This was either through private donations to hospitals, etc., for care of the poor or by individual doctors through the use of a *sliding scale* of fees, whereby the wealthy would pay more in order to support the care of the poor. Prior to the extensive growth of health insurance from the 1940s to the present, this was the customary way in which health care was paid for. Direct payment is still customary for low cost health care items.

II. Provision of Service. The army health service, city hospitals, Indian Health Service, and the British National Health Service all receive an annual budget and in return provide a fixed amount of service (so many hospital beds, clinics, doctors, etc.). The amount of services provided may be more or less adequate. The recipient of care pays nothing directly and perhaps nothing indirectly through taxes. For this reason, this form of service payment is frequently used to provide health care for the poor. It relies largely on the individual doctors employed by the service to decide who is to receive care among eligible population and how much care they receive, based on the doctors' definition of medical need.[1]

---

[1]This is not the same as service benefits, as provided by Blue Cross, Blue Shield, and prepaid groups.

III. Insurance and Prepayment. Individuals make a contractual agreement, either singly or in groups, with an insurer who promises to pay for an agreed-upon range of services under specified conditions. The insurer can pay money directly to the subscriber, or to the provider of services (e.g., Blue Cross, Blue Shield). One device to promote widespread coverage of moderate and high income families is the use of *community rating,* whereby all people in the same area (e.g., state) pay the same monthly premium. Another way to do this is to subsidize premium payments for the poor. A third way is government health insurance (Medicare and Medicaid). This form of payment requires careful specification of risks to be covered so that the insurer can estimate the probable size of his benefit payments. It also is subject to such problems as overutilization of services. If a self-pay patient uses a great many health services, it is his concern. If other members of an insured group use a great many services, it increases each member's premium payments and, therefore, each member is affected by the behavior of others (a phenomenon economists call *externalities*). In contrast, the direct provision of services has a more controllable and predictable budgeted level of expenditure.

The difference between prepayment and insurance: Several different definitions are in use:

1. Blue Cross, Blue Shield, and prepaid group practices (e.g., Kaiser-Permanente, HMOs) are *prepayment plans.* They either contract with providers of service or provide the service themselves (HMOs). In contrast, insurance companies do not contract with providers, but only with subscribers, and rather than providing care, they are said to provide *insurance.* Medicare is separately classified.
2. *Prepayment* is payment in advance for services to be used. An expectant mother may pay her doctor in advance for delivering her baby. There may be no pooling of risk in this case. By this definition, Blue Cross and the insurance companies provide *insurance.* Perhaps Medicare Part A, under this definition, would be, in part, prepayment because the worker pays money for Social Security before he becomes 65 and eligible for benefits.
3. There is no difference between prepayment and insurance. By this definition, Blue Cross and Blue Shield are nonprofit insurance companies.
4. Other special definitions of prepayment include combinations of the following features: service benefits, contract with providers, agreement on charges to subscribers, nonprofit, *first dollar coverage,* coverage of a large proportion of the subscribers' health care costs (comprehensive benefits), etc. This definition is, in effect, similar to (1) since Blue Cross and Kaiser both fit these characteristics and insurance companies do not.

Of these different definitions, (1) and (4) are most frequently used.

IV.   Prepayment Plans, HMOs, Kaiser-Permanente, etc.   These plans combine the provision of service with fixed monthly payments by subscribers and the pooling of risk. They are a combination of II and III, described above.

V.   Charitable Contributions, Endowment Funds, Revenue from Other Miscellaneous Sources Used to Provide Care.

Payment of Physicians

Fee for Service.   A fee is charged the patient for each task or *procedure* performed; with differing fees according to the length and difficulty of the task performed.

> *Sliding Fee Scale.*   Variation in the fee charged, according to the patient's income. The poor paying less and the rich paying more for the same service.
> *Relative Value Scale.*   A listing of procedures performed. Each procedure is given an index number which reflects the relative length and complexity of the task. This index number is then multiplied by a dollar amount to obtain the appropriate fee. The California Relative Value Scale is best known.
> *Usual and Customary Fee.*   The fee for a given procedure that is usually charged by the doctor and other doctors in the area.

Capitation.   A fixed amount of money for a given time period is given to the practitioner for each patient under his/her care, regardless of the amount of care that patient receives. Those patients who sign up with the practitioner to pay for care by capitation constitute that practitioner's *panel* of patients.

> *Closed panel practice* means that the practitioner will only care for patients on his panel. This term has been applied to the prepaid group practices and HMO's.

Salary.   A fixed payment, regardless of the amount of work performed or the number of patients seen.

Other Payment Methods.   Physicians working in group practices or in hospitals are paid in a variety of ways that can be very complex mixes of salary, fee for service, percentages of revenue generated, etc.

Free Services.   Practitioners may not charge for care provided. Sometimes a physician on a hospital staff may provide an agreed-upon amount of service in the hospital without pay, in exchange for his hospital admitting privileges.

2. HEALTH INSURANCE AND PREPAYMENT

I. Definition of Insurance and Health Insurance

Insurance can be defined as "protection by written contract against the hazards (in whole or in part) of the happenings of specified fortuitous events."[2]

Health Insurance can be defined as "protection against the costs of hospital and medical care of lost income arising from an illness or injury."

II. Characteristics of Health Insurance Policies

coverage–types of illness, types of treatment for which the policy holder will be recompensed (covered)

age limits–both for new applicants and renewals

exclusions–"specified hazards for which a policy will not provide benefit payments"

benefits–amount of money to be paid for type of illness or treatment

policy term–time period covered by the policy

preexisting conditions–physical conditions of the insured person which existed prior to the issuance of his policy which may or may not be covered

grace period–"a specified time after a policy's premium payment is due in which the protection of the policy continues subject to actual receipt of premium within that time"

rider–an amendment to the policy expanding or decreasing benefits

time limits–the period of time in which notice of claim or proof of loss must be filed in order to obtain benefits

upper limits of coverage–limit set in the policy for maximum payment

waiver–"an agreement attached to a policy which exempts from coverage certain disabilities normally covered by the policy"

Hypothetical Example of a Health Insurance Policy. Hospital (coverage) insurance for people under age 65 (age limit) paying 100 dollars a day (benefits) for each day in the hospital up to fifty days (upper limit of coverage). The policy is good for one year (policy term) and excludes treatment for mental illness and tuberculosis (exclusions). Preexisting medical conditions not covered (preexisting conditions), payments due monthly by the fifth day of the month (five-day grace period), and the company must receive notice of hospitalization not less than thirty days after admission to the hospital (time limit).

---

[2]Quotations from Health Insurance Institute *Source Book of Health Insurance Data* New York, Yearly.

III. More Characteristics of Health
     Insurance Policies

Premium—"the periodic payment required to keep the policy in force"

Indemnity—"a benefit paid by a health insurance policy for an insured loss"

Claim—"a demand by an insured person for benefits provided by a policy"—a request for payment

Non-Cancellable (Guaranteed Renewable) Policy—(Opposite of an "optional renewable policy") "a policy which the insured has the right to continue in force by the timely payment of premiums set forth in the policy to a specified age during which period the insurer has no right to make any change in any provision of the policy while the policy is in force." Usually, the insurer can not change the premium rate for an individual insured person. The insurer may or may not be allowed to make premium rate changes for all similar policyholders.

Group Insurance (as distinct from *Individual* or *Personal Insurance*)—"a policy protecting a group of persons—usually employees for a firm," rather than a policy providing protection to a policyholder and/or family. One difference is that the insurer estimates the expected risk for the group as a whole, rather than for each individual.

IV. Other Types of Benefits

Coinsurance—a policy provision by which both the insured person and the insurance company share the expenses of illness or injury in a specified proportion. (For example, the insurer will pay 80 percent of the hospital bill while the insured pays the remaining 20 percent.)

Deductible—"that portion of covered hospital and medical charges which the insured person must pay before benefits begin." This is in contrast to *first dollar coverage,* where there is no deductible.

Assignment of Benefits (Non-Service Benefits)—Frequently hospitals or other providers of care will have patients assign (transfer) the benefits from the patient to the hospital so that the insurance company pays the hospital directly.

V. Community vs. Experience Rating of Premiums

In *community rating,* all the people in an area (e.g., a state) would pay the same premium, whether they are young or old, rich or poor, and in spite of the fact that some people have a predictably greater chance of using health care benefits. In theis way the high users would not have to pay very high premiums.

In *experience rating,* individuals or groups are charged premiums proportional to their expected level of utilization.

Under competitive conditions, community rating is not possible because other insurers will offer lower premiums to low risk groups, leaving the community rating insurer with the high risk groups.

Multiple Coverage is when an individual has more than one insurance or prepayment policy covering the same event. In this case, he would make money if the event occurred, and therefore there is a question of moral hazard.

Hypothetical Example of Deductible, Coinsurance, Upper Limit and Not Covered Expenses. The hospital bill is $1,000. The insurance policy has a $100 deductible, 20 percent coinsurance and an upper limit of $600. Three hundred dollars of the hospital bill is not covered because of exclusions in the policy (uninsured expenses[3]). Diagrammatically this can be represented as follows:

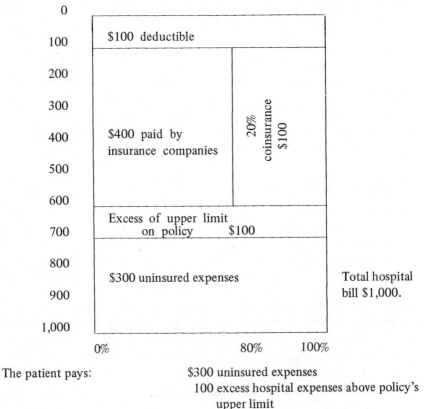

The patient pays:
$300 uninsured expenses
100 excess hospital expenses above policy's upper limit
100 deductible

This leaves $500 of which the company pays 80 percent ($400) and the insured pays 20 percent ($100) through a coinsurance agreement. Thus the company pays $400 and the total bill is $1,000.

---

[3]Figures are chosen for ease of calculation, not as typical of policies in use.

Hypothetical Simplified Example of How Premiums Are Calculated.
Assume the policy is to pay $100 a day (benefit) for each day of hospital
care (coverage) for the first 50 days for each admission (upper limit) for
the coming year (policy term). It is to cover the 1,000 employees of
X Company. The company will pay half the cost and the employees will
have the other half deducted from their monthly pay check. By analyzing
the previous year's experience of these employees it was found that the
average employee used 1.1 hospital days per year, or 1,100 total days
for all 1,000 employees. It was also found that the total number of hospital
days in excess of the 50 limit was 100 days.

This leaves 1,000 days of hospital care to be covered at $100 a
day, or $100,000 yearly in total benefits. To this figure is added 20 percent
for administrative expenses, overhead, reserves, profits and so forth, for a
total needed revenue of $120,000 per year. Of this the company pays half,
$60,000, and each individual employee pays $60 per year or $5 per month—the
monthly premium. Modifications in the benefits would make these calculations
much more complex.

VI. Major Forms of Health Insurance

1. hospital (pays hospital bills)
2. surgical (pays for doctor's operating fees and related care)
3. regular medical (pays for nonsurgical doctor fees in hospital and non-
   hospital physician care
4. major medical (pays for all expenses with coinsurance and deductible
   designed especially to cover major illness)
5. disability (loss of income)

VII. Characteristics of the Insured Event

A major problem for insurers and providers is to make their
obligations both predictable and bounded by some upper known limit. The
actuaries who design insurance and benefits (and prepayment, as in Blue Cross)
consider the following characteristics of the event to be covered. These
characteristics play a basic role in defining the extent and type of coverage:

1. The Insured Event should be *unpredictable* or random in the individual
   case but predictable on average. For example, one cannot predict whether
   an individual coin toss will come up heads or not, but one does know that
   there is a 50 percent chance of this happening over many tosses. Thus,
   the concept of pooling of risks. If the event were predictable, then
   one would buy insurance on the day of the event and let the policy
   lapse the day after. (For example, maternity benefits to already pregnant
   mothers.)

2. The Insured Event should be *definable* so that everyone can agree that it has occurred. For example, a broken leg is definable, but it is not so easy to say when a neurosis calls for psychotherapy.

3. The Insured Event should be *uncontrollable,* like lightning striking a barn. To the extent that events are controllable there is the issue of *moral hazard;* for example, the owner of a failing company who sets fire to the building in order to collect the fire insurance. Because of this problem, insurance usually pays less than the real value of the total loss. In health insurance there is the possible moral hazard of doctors and patients conspiring to use unnecessary health care.

4. The Insured Event should be relatively *large* so that the *administrative costs* of writing the insurance coverage are proportionally small. People have enough money available to cover small events. It is the big costs which may bankrupt them. One reason for a deductible is to avoid the administrative costs of processing small claims.

5. Insured Events should be *independent* events in the statistical sense. Non-independent events are the plague, war, and widespread natural disasters where, if one person is harmed, many others will also be harmed. The large expenditures that would result would bankrupt the insurance company.

6. Expenses connected with the event should be *finite,* known and defined. This allows the insurer to estimate how much he can expect to pay out, and that payments will not be infinitely large. For this reason most insurance policies have upper limits on coverage and some arrangement to insure that they do not have to pay if the doctor charges a very high fee or if the automobile repairman submits an inflated bill.

7. The average predicted value of the Insured Event occurring is small enough so that people will buy the insurance. Insuring 90-year-old men who have already had two heart attacks for $100,000 in event of their death is an example. If they have a 50 percent chance of dying within the year, the premium would be $50,000 excluding administrative costs.

The more the event is characterized by the above, the more appropriate the insurance approach.

In short, insurance is the pooling of risks, but when the insurance company undertakes to cover a risk, it, too, wants to set predictable limits on its commitments.[4]

---

[4]*Reinsurance* is insuring the insurance company against too great a loss. For example, having the government undertake to pay for an insurer's yearly benefits if they exceed an agreed-upon limit beyond which the insurer, if he had to pay it by himself, would go bankrupt.

One should also distinguish between health insurance and the issue of the equitable distribution of health care (access to health care), i.e., the young paying for the health costs of the old, and the well-to-do paying for the poor.

VIII. Provision of Services

This approach, unlike the insurance approach to defining risk above, is to provide a certain fixed level of services for a given population, to be used up to a limit. If there is demand or need in excess of services provided, people may either wait for care (*queue*) or go without. Urban city hospitals for the care of the poor are an example of this approach.

IX. Providers of Private Insurance
(Non-government Agencies)

Blue Cross—"an independent (nongovernment, private) non-profit tax-exempt membership corporation providing protection against the costs of hospital care in a limited geographic area"

Blue Shield—"an independent nonprofit membership corporation providing protection against the costs of surgery and other items of medical care in a limited geographic area"

Blue Cross and Blue Shield (the Blues, or BC-BS, or BX) are legally independent of each other, but often work in close cooperation with each other in offering matched benefit packages to insured groups.

There are approximately seventy Blue Cross organizations covering part of a state (Associated Hospital Service of New York), an entire state (Massachusetts Blue Cross), or several states (Vermont and New Hampshire).

They are linked as members of the Blue Cross Association which provides shared services and arranges for coverage with other Blue Cross plans for travelers who leave their own plan's area.

Blue Cross is set up in most states under special enabling legislation, generally providing that it should be regulated by the state insurance department. In some states Blue Cross must submit to public hearings before it can raise its rates.

Up to 1972 the American Hospital Association owned the Blue Cross symbol and set requirements for corporations using this symbol, including (a) it cover a large enough area, (b) provide service benefits, (c) should have a contract with the majority of hospitals in its area, and (d) have at least one-third of the board representing the public and one-third representing the contracting hospitals.

Blue Cross calls these features which distinguish it from other

private insurance companies "prepayment" rather than "insurance." *Service benefits* (as opposed to direct (cash) payments to insured persons to pay for care, which are called *indemnity benefits*) consist of "a contract benefit which is paid directly to the provider of hospital or medical care for services rendered."

This requires a contractual agreement between the insurer and provider of care (hospitals and Blue Cross, doctors and Blue Shield) and distinguishes the Blue Cross, Blue Shield plans from the commercial insurers who make payments to the (beneficiary) patient, not the provider.

The Blue Cross contract usually specifies what the hospital is allowed to charge the patients covered by Blue Cross. The hospitals are not limited in this way with patients covered by commercial insurance policies.

Blue Cross Enabling Legislation at the State Level. Although the contents of this legislation varies from state to state, it usually includes the following:

a. Blue Cross and Blue Shield are allowed to operate in the state.
b. The state insurance commissioner is given certain powers to regulate the plan.
c. Premium rate increases must be approved by the insurance commissioner after a public hearing.
d. Blue Cross and Blue Shield are the only organizations which are allowed to contract with providers for service benefits at agreed-upon charges.

Private Insurance Companies[5]
Several hundred companies write health insurance, using thousands of different policies. Some major companies include Prudential, Equitable, Aetna, Metropolitan, and Connecticut General.

Independent (Private Insurance) Plans
These plans include:

Kaiser-Permanente Plan
Health Insurance Plan of Greater New York (HIP)
Various union-sponsored plans

These are generally in the form of prepaid group practice.

Workmen's Compensation
Started in the first decade of this century. By 1948 all states had workmen's compensation, in addition to the Federal Employees Compensation

[5]These are sometimes called *commercial insurance companies.* The word "commercial" is not used by the companies in this category and has ideological implications related to the competition between these companies and Blue Cross and Blue Shield.

Act (FECA, passed in 1908, replaced in 1916, and amended in 1949 by PL 81-357), and the Longshoremen and Harbor Workers Act. These laws are based on the idea that the employer is financially liable for injuries to employees, although the employee does not have to prove that the employer was negligent.

There are three categories of benefits:

a. cash,
b. medical, and
c. rehabilitation

to indemnify the worker injured on the job or his dependents for loss of wages, medical and hospital expenses, and loss of occupational capacity and skills.

These benefits are financed by employers, either through insuring with a private insurance company or, in some states, through a state fund or by self-insurance. Benefits vary substantially from state to state and by type of employment.

References

Health Insurance Institute, *Source Book of Health Insurance Data,* New York, Yearly (Quotations from this source).

American Hospital Association, *Approval Program for Blue Cross Plans* (Chicago: The Association, 1964).

Health/PAC Bulletin, "Health Research Guide," New York, No. 28, February 1971.

O. D. Dickerson, *Health Insurance* (Homewood, Illinois: Richard D. Irwin, Inc., 1959).

H. M. Somers and A. R. Somers, *Workman's Compensation* (New York: John Wiley & Sons, 1954).

3. HEALTH PLANS, HMOs

Health plans include *Health Maintenance Organizations* (HMOs) and *Prepaid Group Practice* (PGP). HMO is the more general term. In fact, it is often so general as to be difficult to define. HMOs include Prepaid Group Practice and *Foundations for Medical Care* (FMC), which are described under ambulatory care.

Characteristics of HMOs include the following:

1. It provides directly, or through arrangement with other health services, to enrollees on a per capita prepayment basis. Thus it has a defined population

being served. Each enrollee pays a fixed amount, regardless of the volume of services he uses.

2. The HMO provides physician services through physicians who are partners or employees, or through a contractual arrangement with a group of physicians.
3. The services provided are comprehensive, that is, covering a range of services, usually including inpatient and outpatient care.
4. There are internal, self-regulating mechanisms to assure quality of care and cost control. An organization is responsible for the health care of the population served.

Thus, HMOs combine the provision of service, the barring or risk (insurance or prepayment), and performance monitoring. For many people, one of the ideas behind HMOs is that HMO doctors will be responsible for the hospital bill incurred when they admit a patient to the hospital and, therefore, the HMO doctors will be careful not to admit patients unnecessarily.

Prepaid Group Practice or *Comprehensive Prepaid Group Practice* refers to an HMO where services are provided by doctors in organized group practice. PGPs may or may not own their own hospitals. (For example, Kaiser does and GHI and HIP do not.)

Some of the well-known PGPs include

GHI (Group Health Association of Washington, D.C.)
Group Health Cooperative of Puget Sound (Washington)
Harvard Community Health Plan (Boston)
HIP (Health Insurance Plan of Greater New York)
HMO International (Los Angeles)
Kaiser-Permanente
Ross-Loos Medical Group (Los Angeles)

Although it has many distinctive features when compared with other plans, Kaiser-Permanente, the largest and most frequently cited example, will be described here.

Kaiser-Permanente

This is the largest, nongovernmental *prepaid group practice* health plan in the country. Permanente Medical Groups and the Kaiser Foundation Hospitals are two separate corporate entities working closely together to provide

a. a nongovernment (private),
b. prepaid (fixed monthly payments by members regardless of use of services),
c. group practice (three or more doctors practicing together and sharing income),
d. nonprofit,

e. comprehensive health plan (provides a wide range of doctor, hospital and ancillary services) serving an identifiable population (consumer groups and individuals).

The plan was started to take care of the employees of Kaiser Industries prior to World War II and was opened to the public just after the war. By 1970 it served 2.1 million members in California, Oregon, Washington, Hawaii, Colorado, and Ohio. Most members are enrolled according to their place of employment (group employment).

Physicians are members or partners of the Permanente Medical Groups. The Kaiser Foundation Hospitals own and operate their facilities. Emphasis is placed on outpatient rather than inpatient services. Doctors' offices are usually in or near the hospital and physicians are salaried. In some parts of Kaiser-Permanente, part of any surplus revenue generated by the plan is returned to physicians so there is a financial incentive here for them to keep total costs down. The plan has a lower admission rate per 1,000 population to hospitals in comparison to adjacent Blue Cross–Blue Shield subscribers.

References

Greer Williams, *Kaiser-Permanente Health Plan: Why It Works* (The Henry Kaiser Foundation, 300 Lakeside Drive, Oakland, California 94604, 1971).

Report of the National Advisory Commission on Health Manpower (Washington, D.C.: U.S. Government Printing Office, November 1967), Vol. II, Appendix IV.

"Kaiser-Permanente–Controversial Plan in News," *American Medical News,* September 13, 1971.

Anne R. Somers (editor), *The Kaiser-Permanente Medical Care Program: A Symposium* (New York: The Commonwealth Fund, 1971).

4. FINANCING

The Flow of Funds for the Provision of Health Care

Customarily, payments for health insurance and Medicare Part A are made in relationship to place of employment. The employee and employer pay taxes and Social Security payments (employer contribution and employee's *payroll deduction*). Insurance, Blue Cross, or other coverage for the employee and his family (dependents) is also customarily obtained at the place of employment (*employee benefit plans*). The employee pays through payroll deductions and the employer usually contributes to the premium as a *fringe benefit.* (Fringe benefits are non-salary compensations, such as health and life insurance, retirement benefits, etc.) Blue Cross provides payments directly to the provider (vendor) in the form of service benefits. These providers are under contract. Insurance companies have no contractual arrangement with

providers (usually this is forbidden by state insurance laws). Insurance companies pay benefits directly to the subscriber who, in turn, pays the provider. The subscriber may *assign* his benefits to the provider and then the insurance company will send its benefit directly to the provider. In addition, there are *out-of-pocket* (or direct) expenses paid directly by the user to the provider.

Finally, there are some unemployed, uninsured, and/or indigent persons who make no payments for the care they receive.

Government expenditures are (at the federal, state, and local levels) both for services provided (government hospitals, for example) and for payment to non-governmental providers (*vendor payments*). In this context, government, Blue Cross-Blue Shield, and insurance companies are referred to as *third party payers* (the other "parties" being patient and provider).

The agreement between providers (usually hospitals) and third party payers (usually Blue Cross, and government programs) as to what will be paid for and how much is called the *reimbursement formula.* These can be exceedingly complicated. For example, "cost or charges, whichever is less" means that the third party payer will pay either the provider's actual costs, or what it ordinarily charges patients, whichever figure is lower.

Prospective reimbursement means that the payer and the provider agree in advance on a budget for the provider and, therefore, on the provider's expected costs. If the provider's services cost more, then the provider must absorb the loss. If the provider's services cost less, the provider keeps the extra. This, and other formulae which try to encourage efficient provider performance, is called *incentive reimbursement.*

Preadmission (Prospective) Screening of Admissions means that the doctor and/or hospital must receive prior approval from the payer to admit an elective patient, in order to be reimbursed.

Retrospective Denial of Payment means that the payer reviews the appropriateness of the use of services, after they have been used. If the payer finds the services provided were medically unnecessary, it will not reimburse the provider for them.

National Health Expenditure Data

As the charts and tables on pages 92-100 indicate:

1. National health expenditures have been rising and include a growing share of the *gross national product* (the value of all goods and services produced in the country during the year).
2. The proportion of health care expenditures paid by the government has been increasing.
3. Federal health expenditures are greater than state and local expenditures.
4. Type of payment varies by the type of service provided.

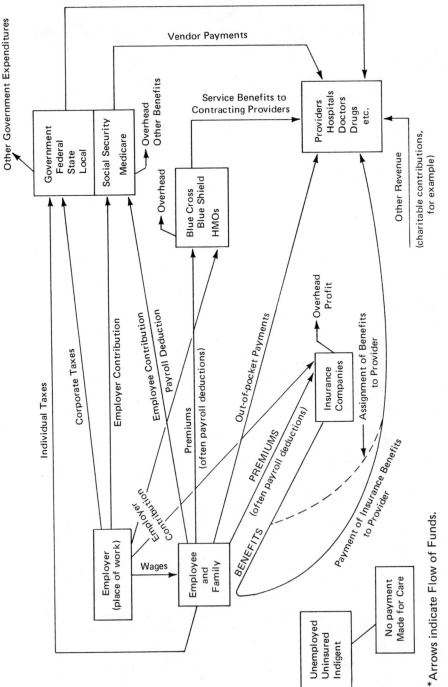

Grants for Research or Special Projects
Payment for Services (Medicaid, for example)
Provision of Services (government hospitals, for example)

Vendor Payments

Other Government Expenditures

Service Benefits to
Contracting Providers

Government
Federal
State
Local

Social Security
Medicare

Overhead
Other Benefits

Providers
Hospitals
Doctors
Drugs
etc.

Overhead

Blue Cross
Blue Shield
HMOs

Other Revenue
(charitable contributions,
for example)

Overhead
Profit

Insurance
Companies

Assignment of Benefits
to Provider

Individual Taxes

Corporate Taxes

Employer Contribution

Employee Contribution
Payroll Deduction

Premiums
(often payroll deductions)

Out-of-Pocket Payments

PREMIUMS
(often payroll deductions)

Payment of Insurance Benefits
to Provider

Employer
Contribution

Employer
(place of work)

Wages

Employee
and
Family

BENEFITS

Unemployed
Uninsured
Indigent

No payment
Made for Care

*Arrows indicate Flow of Funds.

Figure 3-1. Payment for Health Services: Schematic Diagram of Flow of Funds* (Simplified).

Need and Demand for Care

Need for care—This usually refers to an expert estimate of the health services
a person or population requires.

Unmet need—The difference between *realized demand* and *need*

Realized demand—The amount of health care actually used

Demand—(a) Medical care definition: The amount of care that people would
use if there were no barriers to use (like cost or access); (b) Economic
definition: The amount of care purchased at a given price.

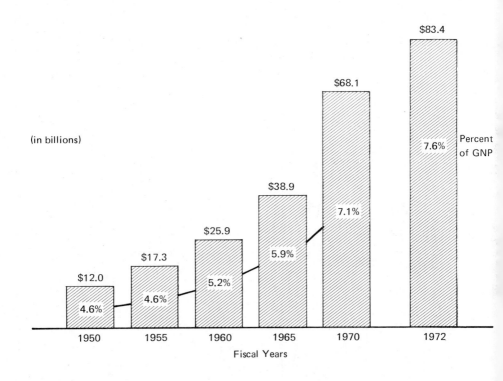

Source: Barbara S. Cooper and Nancy L. Worthington, "National Health
Expenditures 1929–72," *Social Security Bulletin* 36, 1 (January 1973).

Figure 3-2. National Health Expenditures and Percentage of Gross
National Product, Selected Fiscal Years, 1950–72.

Table 3-1. Aggregate and Per Capita National Health Expenditures, by Source of Funds, and Percentage of Gross National Product, Selected Fiscal Years, 1928-29 through 1971-72

Fiscal year	Gross national product (in billions)	Health expenditures								
		Total			Private			Public		
		Amount (in millions)	Per capita	Percent of GNP	Amount (in millions)	Per capita	Percent of total	Amount (in millions)	Per capita	Percent of total
1928-29	$101.0	$3,589	$29.16	3.6	$3,112	$25.28	86.7	$477	$3.88	13.3
1934-35	68.7	2,846	22.04	4.1	2,303	17.84	80.9	543	4.21	19.1
1939-40	95.1	3,863	28.83	4.1	3,081	22.99	79.8	782	5.84	20.2
1949-50	263.4	12,028	78.35	4.6	8,962	58.38	74.5	3,065	19.97	25.5
1954-55	379.7	17,330	103.76	4.6	12,909	77.29	74.5	4,420	26.46	25.5
1959-60	495.6	25,856	141.63	5.2	19,460	106.60	75.3	6,395	35.03	24.7
1964-65	655.6	38,892	197.81	5.9	29,357	149.32	75.5	9,535	48.50	24.5
1965-66	718.5	42,109	211.64	5.9	31,279	157.21	74.3	10,830	54.43	25.7
1966-67	771.4	47,860	237.93	6.2	32,037	159.27	66.9	15,823	78.66	33.1
1967-68	827.0	53,563	263.49	6.5	33,523	164.91	62.6	20,040	98.58	37.4
1968-69	899.0	59,975	292.19	6.7	37,041	180.46	61.8	22,934	111.73	38.2
1969-70	955.1	68,058	328.17	7.1	42,823	206.49	62.9	25,235	121.68	37.1
1970-71	1,010.6	75,624	360.89	7.5	47,048	224.52	62.2	28,576	136.37	37.8
1971-72	1,095.9	83,417	394.16	7.6	50,560	238.90	60.6	32,857	155.25	39.4

Source: Barbara S. Cooper and Nancy L. Worthington, "National Health Expenditures 1929-72," *Social Security Bulletin* 36, 1 (January 1973).

Table 3-2. National Health Expenditures, by Type of Expenditure and Source of Funds, Fiscal Years, 1969-70 through 1971-72 (in millions)

| Type of expenditure | Total | Source of funds | | | | | |
| | | Private | | | Public | | |
		Total	Consumers	Other	Total	Federal	State and local
				1971-72			
Total	$83,417	$50,560	$46,170	$4,390	$32,857	$21,560	$11,297
Health services and supplies	77,291	47,665	46,170	1,495	29,625	19,207	10,418
Hospital care	32,460	15,267	14,840	427	17,193	11,220	5,973
Physician's services	16,150	12,430	12,419	11	3,720	2,803	916
Dentists' services	5,025	4,771	4,771		254	165	90
Other professional services[1]	1,655	1,427	1,395	32	228	166	62
Drugs and drug sundries[1]	7,909	7,340	7,340		569	303	266
Eyeglasses and appliances	2,037	1,960	1,960		77	44	34
Nursing-home care	3,500	1,370	1,345	25	2,130	1,282	848
Expenses for prepayment and administration	2,868	2,100	2,100		768	638	130
Government public health activities	2,100				2,100	823	1,276
Other health services	3,587	1,000		1,000	2,587	1,763	824
Research and medical-facilities construction	6,127	2,895		2,895	3,232	2,353	879
Research[1]	2,029	195		195	1,834	1,755	79
Construction	4,098	2,700		2,700	1,398	598	800
Publicly owned facilities	1,052				1,052	266	786
Privately owned facilities	3,046	2,700		2,700	346	332	14
				1970-71			
Total	$75,624	$47,048	$43,176	$3,872	$28,576	$18,764	$9,812
Health services and supplies	70,182	44,571	43,176	1,395	25,611	16,658	8,952
Hospital care	29,357	14,447	14,047	400	14,910	9,739	5,171
Physicians' services	15,038	11,612	11,601	11	3,426	2,586	840
Dentists' services	4,637	4,402	4,402		235	148	87
Other professional services	1,542	1,341	1,311	30	201	148	53

	Total	Private total	Direct / consumer	Other private	Public total	Federal	State and local
Drugs and drug sundries[1]	7,506	6,988	6,988		518	276	242
Eyeglasses and appliances	1,922	1,856	1,856		66	35	31
Nursing-home care	3,282	1,309	1,286	23	1,973	1,196	777
Expenses for prepayment and administration	2,383	1,685	1,685		698	569	129
Government public health activities	1,698				1,698	678	1,021
Other health services	2,817	931		931	1,886	1,283	603
Research and medical-facilities construction	5,443	2,477		2,477	2,966	2,106	860
Research[1]	1,838	195		195	1,643	1,565	78
Construction	3,605	2,282		2,282	1,323	541	782
Publicly owned facilities	909				909	141	768
Privately owned facilities	2,696	2,282		2,282	414	400	14
Total	**$68,058**	**$42,823**	**$39,174**	**$3,649**	**$25,235**	**$16,598**	**$8,637**

1969-70

	Total	Private total	Direct / consumer	Other private	Public total	Federal	State and local
Health services and supplies	63,044	40,464	39,174	1,290	22,579	14,492	8,087
Hospital care	25,929	12,997	12,626	371	12,932	8,283	4,648
Physicians' services	13,447	10,324	10,314	10	3,123	2,378	745
Dentists' services	4,233	4,029	4,029		204	114	89
Other professional services	1,386	1,176	1,149	27	210	155	55
Drugs and drug sundries[1]	7,057	6,613	6,613		444	221	224
Eyeglasses and appliances	1,814	1,755	1,755		59	31	29
Nursing-home care	2,860	1,195	1,173	22	1,665	1,001	604
Expenses for prepayment and administration	2,105	1,515	1,515		590	491	98
Government public health activities	1,437				1,437	590	847
Other health services	2,776	860		860	1,916	1,228	688
Research and medical-facilities construction	5,015	2,359		2,359	2,656	2,106	550
Research[1]	1,846	193		193	1,659	1,577	76
Construction	3,169	2,166		2,166	1,003	529	474
Publicly owned facilities	820				820	359	461
Privately owned facilities	2,319	2,166		2,166	183	170	13

[1] Research expenditures-of drug companies included in drugs and drug sundries and excluded from research expenditures.

Source: Barbara S. Cooper and Nancy L. Worthington, "National Health Expenditures 1929-72," *Social Security Bulletin* 36, 1 (January 1973).

Table 3-3.   Expenditures for Health Services and Supplies under Public Programs, by Program, Type of Expenditures, and Source of Funds, Fiscal Year 1971-72. (in millions)

Program and source of funds	Total	Hospital care	Physicians' services	Dentists' services	Other professional services	Drugs and drug sundries	Eye-glasses and appliances	Nursing-home care	Government public health activities	Other health services	Administration
					1971-72						
Total	$29,624.8	$17,192.9	$3,719.6	$254.5	$227.5	$569.0	$77.2	$2,129.8	$2,099.7	$2,586.6	$767.7
Health insurance for the aged[1,2]	8,819.2	6,017.1	2,006.1		82.0			216.0		43.0	455.0
Temporary disability insurance (medical benefits)[3]	74.2	53.7	17.6		1.2	.8	.8				
Workmen's compensation (medical benefits)	1,200.0	604.5	510.6		36.9	24.0	24.0				
Public assistance (vendor medical payments)[2]	7,602.7	3,207.0	781.2	185.0	34.3	513.9		1,822.8		768.2	290.2
General hospital and medical care	4,235.4	4,181.4	7.4	1.7		1.3				43.5	
Defense Department hospital and medical care including military dependents[4]	2,187.8	1,393.4	155.2						639.2		
Maternal and child health services	499.2	74.7	44.7	11.1	36.0	10.7	14.3			307.7	
School health	295.0									295.0	
Other public health activities	2,099.7								2,099.7		
Veterans' hospital and medical care[4]	2,255.6	1,592.1	18.4	47.9		4.1	19.7	91.0		459.9	22.5
Medical vocational rehabilitation	179.1	69.0	91.7				18.4				
Office of Economic Opportunity	176.9		86.7	8.8	37.1	14.2				30.1	
Federal	19,206.9	11,220.2	2,803.3	164.8	165.7	302.9	43.5	1,282.1	823.2	1,763.1	637.9
Health insurance for the aged[1,2]	8,819.2	6,017.1	2,006.1		82.0			216.0		43.0	455.0
Workmen's compensation (medical benefits)	30.0	19.5	7.5		1.8	.6	.6				
Public assistance (vendor medical payments)[2]	4,089.9	1,715.5	417.9	99.0	18.3	274.9		975.1		428.7	160.4

General hospital and medical care	446.3		7.4	1.7		1.3				43.5	
Defense Department hospital and medical care (including military dependents)[4]	392.3			7.4						639.2	
Maternal and child health services	2,187.8	1,393.4	155.2	26.5		7.8	8.5			118.7	
Other public health activities	234.7	35.1	30.7					823.2			
Veterans' hospital and medical care[4]	2,255.6	1,692.1	18.4	47.9		4.1	19.7			459.9	22.5
Medical vocational rehabilitation	143.3	55.2	73.4	8.8				91.0		30.1	
Office of Economic Opportunity	176.9		86.7	37.1		14.2	14.7				
State and local	10,418.0	5,972.7	916.3	89.7	61.7	266.1	33.7	847.7	1,276.5	823.5	129.8
Temporary disability insurance (medical benefits)[3]	74.2	53.7	17.6	1.2		.8	.8				
Workmen's compensation (medical benefits)	1,170.0	585.0	503.1	35.1		23.4	23.4				
Public assistance (vendor medical payments)[2]	3,512.9	1,491.5	363.3	15.9	86.0	239.0		847.7		339.5	129.8
General hospital and medical care	3,789.1		3,789.1	3.7							
Maternal and child health services	264.5	39.6	14.0	9.5		2.9	5.8			189.0	
School health	295.0			3.7						295.0	
Other public health activities	1,276.5									1,276.5	
Medical vocational rehabilitation	35.8	13.8	18.3				3.7				

[1] Includes premium payments for supplementary medical insurance by or in behalf of enrollees.

[2] Includes duplication in the Medicare and Medicaid amount where premium payments for Medicare are paid for by Medicaid for old-age recipients and, in some States, for the aged medically indigent.

[3] Includes medical benefits paid under public law by private insurance carriers and self-insurers.

[4] Payments for services outside the hospital (excluding "other health services") represent only those made under contract medical care programs.

Source: Barbara S. Cooper and Nancy L. Worthington, "National Health Expenditures 1929-72," *Social Security Bulletin* 36, 1 (January 1973).

Table 3-4. Aggregate and Per Capita National Health Expenditures, by Type of Expenditure, Selected Fiscal Years, 1928-29 through 1971-72

Type of expenditure	1928-29	1934-35	1939-40	1949-50	1954-55	1959-60	1964-65	1965-66	1966-67	1967-68	1968-69	1969-70	1970-71	1971-72
							Aggregate amount (in millions)							
Total	$3,589	$2,846	$3,863	$12,028	$17,330	$25,856	$38,892	$42,109	$47,860	$53,563	$59,975	$68,058	$75,624	$83,417
Health services and supplies	3,382	2,788	3,729	11,181	16,392	24,162	35,664	38,661	44,324	49,599	55,686	63,044	70,182	77,291
Hospital care	651	731	969	3,698	5,689	8,499	13,152	14,245	16,921	19,384	22,356	25,929	29,357	32,460
Physicians' services	994	744	946	2,689	3,632	5,580	8,405	8,865	9,738	10,734	11,842	13,447	15,038	16,150
Dentists' services	476	298	402	940	1,457	1,944	2,728	2,866	3,158	3,498	3,821	4,233	4,637	5,025
Other professional services	248	150	173	384	552	848	989	1,140	1,139	1,210	1,292	1,386	1,542	1,655
Drugs and drug sundries	601	471	624	1,642	2,282	3,591	4,647	5,032	5,480	5,864	6,480	7,057	7,506	7,909
Eyeglasses and appliances	131	128	180	475	605	750	1,151	1,309	1,514	1,665	1,743	1,814	1,992	2,037
Nursing-home care			28	178	291	480	1,271	1,407	1,692	2,070	2,465	2,860	3,282	3,500
Expenses for prepayment and administration	101	91	161	290	605	807	1,234	1,446	1,820	1,935	2,058	2,105	2,383	2,868
Government public health activities	89	112	155	351	384	401	671	731	884	1,001	1,195	1,437	1,698	2,100
Other health services	90	63	92	534	895	1,262	1,416	1,620	1,978	2,238	2,434	2,776	2,817	3,587
Research and medical-facilities construction	207	58	134	847	938	1,694	3,228	3,448	3,536	3,964	4,290	5,015	5,443	6,127
Research			3	110	194	592	1,391	1,545	1,606	1,800	1,790	1,846	1,838	2,029

Construction	207	58	131	737	744	1,102	1,837	1,903	1,930	2,164	2,500	3,169	3,605	4,098
							Per capita amount[1]							
Total	$29.16	$22.04	$28.83	$78.35	$103.76	$141.63	$197.81	$211.64	$237.93	$263.49	$292.19	$328.17	$360.89	$394.16
Health services and supplies	27.48	21.59	27.83	72.83	98.14	132.35	181.39	194.31	220.35	243.99	271.29	303.99	334.92	365.21
Hospital care	5.29	5.66	7.23	24.09	34.06	46.56	66.89	71.59	84.12	95.35	108.91	125.03	140.10	153.38
Physicians' services	8.08	5.76	7.06	17.52	21.75	30.57	42.75	44.56	48.41	52.80	57.69	64.84	71.76	76.31
Dentists' services	3.87	2.31	3.00	6.12	8.72	10.65	13.88	14.40	15.70	17.21	18.62	20.41	22.13	23.74
Other professional services	2.01	1.16	1.29	2.50	3.30	4.65	5.03	5.73	5.66	5.95	6.29	6.68	7.36	7.82
Drugs and drug sundries	4.88	3.65	4.66	10.70	13.66	19.67	23.64	25.29	27.24	28.85	31.57	34.03	35.82	37.37
Eyeglasses and appliances	1.06	.99	1.34	3.09	3.62	4.11	5.85	6.58	7.53	8.19	8.49	8.75	9.17	9.63
Nursing-home care		.21	.21	1.16	1.74	2.63	6.46	7.07	8.41	10.18	12.01	13.79	15.66	16.54
Expenses for prepayment and administration	.82	.70	1.20	1.89	3.62	4.42	6.28	7.27	9.05	9.52	10.03	10.15	11.37	13.55
Government public health activities	.72	.87	1.16	2.29	2.30	2.19	3.41	3.67	4.39	4.92	5.82	6.93	8.10	9.92
Other health services	.73	.49	.69	3.48	5.36	6.91	7.20	8.14	9.83	11.01	11.86	13.39	13.44	16.95
Research and medical-facilities construction	1.68	.45	1.00	5.52	5.62	9.28	16.42	17.33	17.58	19.50	20.90	24.28	25.98	28.95
Research			.02	.72	1.16	3.24	7.07	7.77	7.98	8.85	8.72	8.90	8.77	9.59
Construction	1.68	.45	.98	4.80	4.45	6.04	9.34	9.56	9.59	10.65	12.18	15.28	17.20	19.36

[1] Based on January 1 data from the Bureau of the Census for total U.S. population (including Armed Forces and Federal civilian employees overseas and the civilian population of outlying areas).

Source: Barbara S. Cooper and Nancy L. Worthington, "National Health Expenditures 1929-72," *Social Security Bulletin* 36, 1 (January 1973).

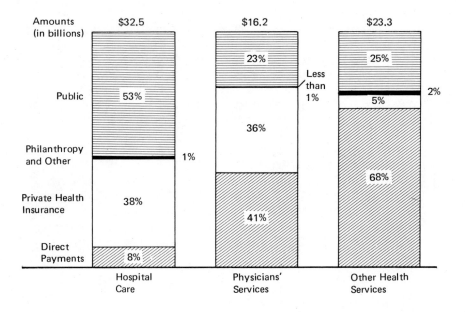

Source: Barbara S. Cooper and Nancy L. Worthington, "National Health Expenditures 1929-72," *Social Security Bulletin* 36, 1 (January 1973).

Figure 3-3. Distribution of Personal Health Care Expenditures, by Source of Funds and Type of Expenditures, Fiscal Year 1972.

Chapter Four

The Federal Government and Health Care

1. THE FEDERAL GOVERNMENT AND HEALTH: OVERVIEW

There is no constitutionally defined role for the federal government in health and therefore such activities have been traditionally reserved to the states. Nevertheless, there has been over the years a gradual development of a federal presence in the field of health. The routes of this still expanding role include:

a. the special responsibility for certain population groups, such as merchant seamen, members of the armed forces, veterans, and American Indians;
b. responsibilities in the areas of foreign and interstate relationships, such as immigration and quarantine, and the regulation of food and drugs and safety standards;[1]
c. grants-in-aid to states, institutions and individuals for a wide variety of activities;
d. most recently, sponsorship and financial participation in the health insurance program for the elderly (Medicare).

Many of the federal health-related functions are consolidated in the Department of Health, Education and Welfare (see Section 2, below), Many, however, are among the responsibilities of a variety of other departments, agencies, and bureaus, where they generally represent only a part of or are incidental to the main activities of the unit. The more important of these are briefly noted on the following pages.[2]

---

[1] Much of the regulatory power of the federal government in health, as in other areas, derives from the constitutional power to regulate interstate commerce.

[2] A more complete list, as of 1969, may be found in *Principles of Public Health Administration* by John J. Hanlon (Saint Louis: C. V. Moseley Company, 1969), p. 225.

Executive Office of the President

Office of Management and Budget. This office was organized in 1970, replacing the *Bureau of the Budget*. It is responsible for the preparation, supervision and control of the federal budget and for the overall administration and management of the Executive Branch. This agency thus greatly affects the operation and activities of all federal agencies.

Office of Economic Opportunity. This office is responsible for the administration and coordination of federal antipoverty programs under the Economic Opportunity Act of 1964. Its *Office of Health Affairs* administers the health-related functions.

Special Action Office for Drug Abuse Prevention. This office was established in 1971 for overall planning and coordination of federal drug abuse prevention programs.

Department of Agriculture

This department's activities include responsibility for inspection of meat and poultry, and for food and nutrition programs including food stamps, surplus food, and child nutrition.[3]

Department of Defense

The department is responsible for the health and medical care of members of the armed forces through the *Deputy Assistant Secretary for Health and Environment*. A complete range of health and medical care programs, institutions and training programs is operated.

Civilian medical care for dependents of servicemen is administered through the CHAMPUS insurance program.[4]

Recent legislation has authorized the establishment of an armed forces medical school.[5]

Department of Housing and Urban Development

This department's programs of assistance for urban development and improvement, especially in low income areas, include provision for the improvement of neighborhood health services. In particular, health-related activities are features of many *Model Cities* programs.[6]

---

[3]The child nutrition programs include the National School Lunch Program and the National School Breakfast Program, under the National School Lunch Act of 1946, and the Child Nutrition Act of 1966.

[4]Civilian Health and Medical Program of the Uniformed Services, established under the Dependents Medical Care Act of 1956.

[5]Uniformed Services Revitalization Act of 1972.

[6]"Model Cities" programs have been developed in many urban areas under the Demonstration Cities and Metropolitan Development Act of 1966.

Department of the Interior

This department's *Bureau of Mines* is responsible for control of health and safety hazards in the mining industry.

Department of Labor

This department's *Occupational Safety and Health Administration* is responsible for the promotion of industrial health and safety and the enforcement of related laws and regulations.[7]

Independent Agencies

There are many federal agencies which are not part of Cabinet departments or the Executive Office. They include a wide variety of administrations, agencies, boards, commissions, councils, etc. Among those with some health-related activities are the following.

ACTION. This agency was established in 1971 to incorporate a number of national volunteer programs, including the Peace Corps, VISTA,[8] the Foster Grandparent Program, and the Retired Senior Volunteer Program.

Appalachian Regional Commission. This commission was created in 1965 by the Appalachian Redevelopment Act. It consists of a representative of each of 13 eastern states,[9] a federal co-chairman and a state governor (in rotation) as co-chairman. The purpose of the Commission is to promote the economic and social development of the region. The Commission sponsors a variety of health projects, including community health clinics and manpower training programs.

Environmental Protection Agency. This agency was established in 1970 to coordinate and consolidate federal activities in environmental quality control. Its responsibilities include implementation of the Clean Air Act and the Federal Water Pollution Control Act.

United States Civil Service Commission. The Commission administers the *Federal Employees Health Benefits Programs,* by contracting with health insurance organizations for health benefit plans.[10]

---

[7]The department's activities in this area were considerably expanded by the Occupational Safety and Health Act of 1970.

[8]Volunteers in Service to America; transferred from the Office of Economic Opportunity.

[9]The Appalachian region, for purposes of the Commission, includes portions of: Alabama, Georgia, Kentucky, Maryland, Mississippi, New York, North Carolina, Ohio, Pennsylvania, South Carolina, Tennessee, Virginia, and West Virginia.

[10]This program was established by the Federal Employees Health Benefits Act of 1959.

Veterans Administration. The Veterans Administration's *Department of Medicine and Surgery* administers the program of medical services for veterans of the armed forces who have service-related illnesses and disabilities, or are medically indigent. Services are rendered through an extensive network of V.A. hospitals, clinics, nursing home and residential units, as well as non-V.A. facilities and practitioners. These services are supported by a variety of related manpower training activities including an extensive internship and residency program.

Advisory Groups

There are many advisory groups which have been established for various levels of government. Of special interest are the following.

Advisory Commission on Intergovernmental Relations. This is a 26-member body established by Congress in 1959 to provide a continuing review of the federal system as it relates to state and local governments. Its membership represents federal, state, and local government and the general public. The Commission publishes annual reports which are of considerable general interest.

Advisory Councils. There are many advisory councils which have been established to advise specific government agencies on various matters including policy, regulations and research grant approval. Examples are the Federal Hospital Council (for the Hill-Burton health facilities construction program) and the advisory councils to the several institutes of the National Institutes of Health.

Quasi-Official Agencies

There are a number of agencies which, while not formally a part of the federal government, have a special statutory relationship to it. These include the *National Academy of Sciences*[11] (with the National Research Council and the recently organized Institute of Medicine) and the *American National Red Cross.*[12]

2. THE DEPARTMENT OF HEALTH, EDUCATION AND WELFARE

Historical Note

The Department of Health, Education and Welfare was created in 1953 by elevating to cabinet status the *Federal Security Agency,* which included most of the federal health, education and social welfare agencies functioning

---

[11]Established by an Act of Congress in 1863.

[12]Founded by Clara Barton (1882) and chartered under an Act of Congress in 1863.

at that time.[13] These included the Public Health Service, Food and Drug Administration, Social Security Administration (with the Children's Bureau), Office of Education and the Office of Vocational Rehabilitation (see Table 4-1).

Table 4-1. Department of Health, Education, and Welfare, 1953*

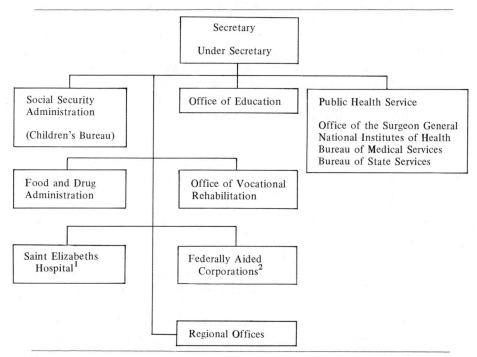

Notes:
1. A psychiatric hospital for residents of the District of Columbia and persons eligible for care by the Public Health Service or Veterans' Administration.
2. The federally aided corporations are supported in part by federal funds appropriated in the budget of the Department of Health, Education and Welfare. They are:
    American Printing House for the Blind
    Columbia Institute for the Deaf (Kendall School and Gallaudet College)
    Howard University

*Abbreviated

Public Health Service.   The United States Public Health Service was the oldest of HEW's component agencies. It was established by Congress in 1798 as the Marine Hospital Service for the "relief of sick and disabled seamen." This care was financed by monthly contributions of twenty cents from each merchant seaman's wages. The Service was placed in the Treasury Department (where it

---

[13]The Federal Security Agency had been created in 1939 to bring together these activities from several departments and agencies.

remained until 1939), and the tax was collected by the Collector of Customs.[14] Gradually, a number of special *marine hospitals* were constructed in principal ports.

In 1878 the Public Health Service was authorized by Congress to develop recommendations for uniform quarantine laws and regulations in the states and to carry out investigations related to the cause and control of epidemic disease. Thereafter, the functions of the service steadily increased. Notable dates were the following:

1887—A research program was begun with the establishment of the *Hygienic Laboratory* at the Marine Hospital on Staten Island, New York.

1889—The professional personnel of the service were organized in a quasi-military *Commissioned Corps* under the Surgeon General.[15]

1893—The service was given full responsibility for foreign and interstate quarantine.

1902—The service was reorganized and renamed the *Public Health and Marine Hospital Service.* It was given responsibility for licensing and regulating the interstate sale of biological products. The Surgeon General was authorized to call an annual conference of state and territorial health officers.

1912—The service was renamed the United States Public Health Service. In subsequent years, its added responsibilities included the National Leprosarium (Carville, La.), a hospital for the treatment of narcotic addicts (Lexington, Ky.), and a Venereal Disease Control division.

1930—The Hygienic Laboratory was redesignated the *National Institute of Health.*

1935—The Social Security Act's Title VI, administered by the Public Health Service, authorized grants-in-aid to the states for strengthening state and local health departments.

1937—The National Cancer Act created the National Cancer Institute, the first specialty institute in the National Institute of Health.

1939—The service was transferred from the Treasury Department to the newly established *Federal Security Agency.*

1944—The Public Health Service Act of 1944 (see Section 13) revised substantially and brought together in one statute all existing legislation concerning the Public Health Service.

1946—The Communicable Disease Center was established (Atlanta, Ga.). The Census Bureau's Division of Vital Statistics was transferred to the service as the National Office of Vital Statistics.

---

[14]Later on this tax, the first U.S. compulsory sickness insurance, was discontinued and costs were paid from general revenues.

[15]Initially, members of the Corps were physicians. Membership was broadened by Acts of Congress in 1930 and 1944 to include dentists, sanitary engineers and pharmacists; and dieticians, nurses, physical therapists, sanitarians, scientists and veterinarians.

1953—The Federal Security Agency became the *Department of Health, Education and Welfare.*

Food and Drug Administration. The Food and Drug Administration was established in the Department of Agriculture in 1927 to administer the several existing acts relating to the quality and safety of food and drugs. It was transferred to the Federal Security Agency in 1940. Its major legislative base was the Food, Drug and Cosmetic Act, originally passed in 1906 (as the Food and Drug Act) and amended many times thereafter.

Social Security Administration. The Social Security Administration (originally the Social Security Board) administered the titles (sections) of the Social Security Act related to Old Age and Survivors Insurance ("social security"), federal aid to state programs for public assistance ("welfare") and unemployment insurance. This agency also included the important *Children's Bureau.*

Children's Bureau. The Children's Bureau was created within the Department of Labor in 1912 to "investigate and report upon . . . all matters pertaining to the welfare of children and child life . . . ." During the next decade it developed an extensive program of studies, research and distribution of educational material relating to the health and welfare of mothers and children.

1921—The Maternity and Infancy Act (Sheppard–Towner Act) provided grants to the states for promotion of maternal and child health work and greatly expanded the scope and activities of the Bureau. Units for child hygiene activities were subsequently established in many states previously without them.

1929—The Maternity and Infancy Act expired and the activities of the Bureau were subsequently curtailed.

1935—Title V of the Social Security Act provided grants-in-aid to the states for maternal and child health, child welfare, and crippled children. The responsibilities of the Bureau were again greatly increased.

1946—The Children's Bureau was transferred from the Department of Labor to the Social Security Administration in the *Federal Security Agency.*

1943
1949 —The Bureau administered the *Emergency Maternity and Infant Care Program* for dependents of servicemen.

Office of Education. The Office of Education was established in the Department of the Interior in 1867 to gather statistics and facts and to diffuse information concerning education. Added responsibilities included the administration of grants-in-aid to land grant colleges (1890), and grants to the states for vocational rehabilitation programs (1920–1943) and vocational education programs (1933). The Office became part of the Federal Security Agency in 1939.

Office of Vocational Rehabilitation. The Office of Vocational Rehabilitation was established in 1943 to administer an expanded program of grants to the states for vocational rehabilitation of disabled persons.[16]

References
Ralph Chester Williams, *The United States Public Health Service 1798-1950* (Washington, D.C.: Commissioned Officers Association of the United States Public Health Service , 1951).

Functions and activities of the National Government in the Field of Welfare. A Report with Recommendations Prepared for the Commission on Organization of the Executive Branch of Government. The Brookings Institution (U.S. Government Printing Office, 1949). A study of the federal functions and activities as of 1948 in the fields of health, education, employment, public assistance, social security, and recreation.

Recent Reorganizations

The Department of Health, Education and Welfare has been reorganized many times since 1953, a process which is still continuing.

In 1963, the *Welfare Administration* was established to administer the public assistance and related social service programs. The Children's Bureau was also transferred to this agency, as were the Office of Aging and the Office of Juvenile Delinquency and Youth Development.[17] In 1967, the Welfare Administration and the Vocational Rehabilitation Administration were absorbed into the new *Social and Rehabilitation Service.*

In 1968, the Public Health Service was reorganized with the creation of the *Health Services and Mental Health Administration* (HSMHA) to incorporate most of the traditional functions of the Service. The Service was placed under the direction of the Assistant Secretary for Health and Scientific Affairs with the Surgeon General his principal deputy. A new *Consumer Protection and Environmental Health Services* agency was established, incorporating the Food and Drug Administration. This was shortlived, however, the FDA again becoming a separate agency within the Public Health Service in 1969, and most of the other functions of the Environmental Health Service being transferred in 1970 to the newly created independent *Environmental Protection Agency.*

Another noteworthy reorganization involved the Children's Bureau. In 1969, the Bureau was moved from the Social and Rehabilitation Service to the new Office of Child Development.[18] Its health programs were placed in the new Maternal and Child Health Service (HSMHA) and its social service programs were merged with programs for adults in the Social and Rehabilitation Service. The Bureau retained responsibility for overall coordination of maternal

---

[16] Authorized under the Vocational Rehabilitation Act Amendments of 1943.
[17] From the Office of the Secretary of HEW.
[18] In the Office of the Secretary of HEW under the Assistant Secretary for Administration.

and child health programs, and its original mandate to investigate and report upon matters relating to health and welfare of children. The Office of Child Development also now included the *Head Start* program.[19]

The general organization of HEW in 1972 is shown in Table 4-2. The Health Services and Mental Health Administration is shown in Table 4-3.

Beginning in July 1973, the health agencies of the Department of Health, Education and Welfare were again extensively reorganized. The Health Services and Mental Health Administration was replaced by two new units, the *Health Services Administration* and the *Health Resources Administration.* The Center for Disease Control became a separate agency, and the National Institute of Mental Health became part of a new Alcohol, Drug Abuse and Mental Health Administration. Finally, the functions of the Bureau of Health Manpower Education were transferred from NIH to the new Health Resources Administration.

Additional changes were also made in the Office of the Secretary of HEW. Among these was the establishment of the position of Assistant Secretary of Human Development, whose responsibilities include the Office of Child Development, Office of Youth Development, and the Administration on Aging.[20]

Present Organization of HEW

The Department of Health, Education and Welfare now[21] consists of ten operating agencies (Table 4-4). Six are under the rubric of the *Public Health Service.*

Alcohol, Drug Abuse and Mental Health Administration
Center for Disease Control
Food and Drug Administration
Health Resources Administration
Health Services Administration
National Institutes of Health

The other four agencies are:
Social Security Administration
Social and Rehabilitation Service
Office of Education[22]
National Institute of Education[22]

Public Health Service

The Public Health Service is under the direction of the Assistant Secretary for Health. No specific functions have been assigned to the Surgeon

---

[19] Transferred from the Office of Economic Opportunity.

[20] The Administration on Aging was transferred from the Social and Rehabilitation Service subsequent to provisions of the 1973 amendments of the Older Americans Act.

[21] February 1974.

[22] The Office of Education and the National Institute of Education make up the *Division of Education.* The Institute was established under the Education Amendments of 1972.

Table 4-2. Department of Health, Education, and Welfare, 1972.[a]

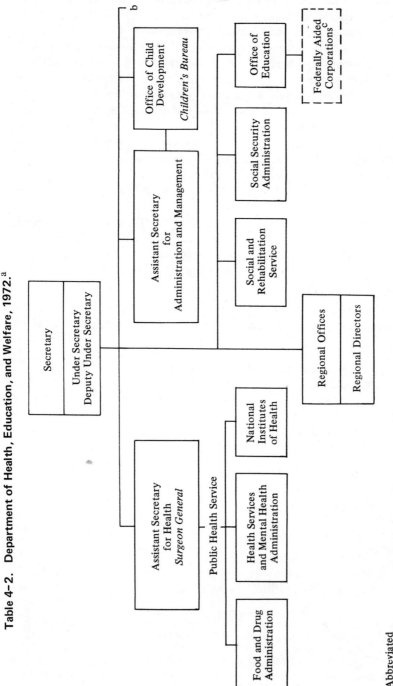

[a]Abbreviated

[b]Also Assistant Secretaries for: Public Affairs, Community and Field Services, Legislation, and Planning and Evaluation.

[c]American Printing House for the Blind, Gallaudet College, Howard University

Table 4-3. Health Services and Mental Health Administration, 1972

Development

    National Center for Health Services
      Research and Development
    Health Care Facilities Service
    Comprehensive Health Planning Service
    Regional Medical Programs Service
    Health Maintenance Organization Service

Health Services Delivery

    National Center for Family Planning
      Services
    Maternal and Child Health Service
    Community Health Service
    Indian Health Service
    Federal Health Programs Service
    National Health Service Corps

Prevention and Consumer Services

    Center for Disease Control
    National Institute of Occupational
      Safety and Health
    Bureau of Community Environmental
    Management

Mental Health

    National Institute of Mental Health
    National Institute on Alcohol Abuse
      and Alcoholism

National Center for Health Statistics

General, and this position is now vacant.[23] The Assistant Secretary's office includes the new Office of Professional Standards Review which has responsibility for professional standards review organization (PSRO) activities.

Alcohol, Drug Abuse and Mental Health Administration

National Institute on Alcohol Abuse and Alcoholism.   This agency is responsible for programs directed toward the problems of alcohol abuse.

National Institute on Drug Abuse.   This agency administers programs directed to the problems of drug abuse.

National Institute of Mental Health.   This agency was established in 1946 as the second specialty institute of the Public Health Service. It was separated from the National Institutes of Health as a separate bureau in 1967, and in 1968 was incorporated into the new Health Services and Mental Health Administration. It administers programs of research, service development and training in mental health, including support of community health centers.

Center for Disease Control (Atlanta).

This is the former National Communicable Disease Center, which was renamed in 1970 when its functions were broadened to include, in addition to its traditional activities related to infectious disease, other preventable conditions including malnutrition.

[23]February 1974.

Table 4–4. Department of Health, Education and Welfare, 1974.[a]

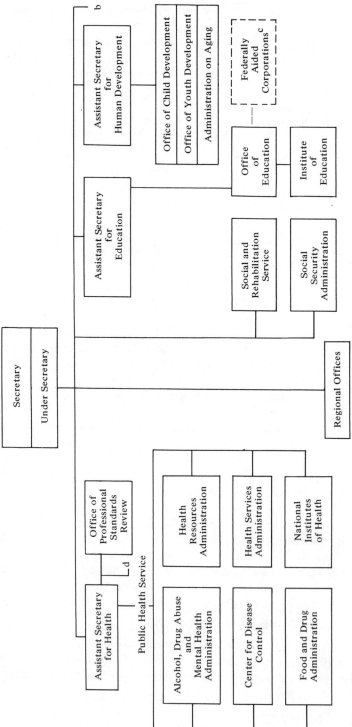

Table 4-3. Health Services and Mental Health Administration, 1972

Development

National Center for Health Services
Research and Development
Health Care Facilities Service
Comprehensive Health Planning Service
Regional Medical Programs Service
Health Maintenance Organization Service

Health Services Delivery

National Center for Family Planning
Services
Maternal and Child Health Service
Community Health Service
Indian Health Service
Federal Health Programs Service
National Health Service Corps

Prevention and Consumer Services

Center for Disease Control
National Institute of Occupational
Safety and Health
Bureau of Community Environmental
Management

Mental Health

National Institute of Mental Health
National Institute on Alcohol Abuse
and Alcoholism

National Center for Health Statistics

General, and this position is now vacant.[23] The Assistant Secretary's office includes the new Office of Professional Standards Review which has responsibility for professional standards review organization (PSRO) activities.

Alcohol, Drug Abuse and Mental Health Administration

National Institute on Alcohol Abuse and Alcoholism. This agency is responsible for programs directed toward the problems of alcohol abuse.

National Institute on Drug Abuse. This agency administers programs directed to the problems of drug abuse.

National Institute of Mental Health. This agency was established in 1946 as the second specialty institute of the Public Health Service. It was separated from the National Institutes of Health as a separate bureau in 1967, and in 1968 was incorporated into the new Health Services and Mental Health Administration. It administers programs of research, service development and training in mental health, including support of community health centers.

Center for Disease Control (Atlanta).

This is the former National Communicable Disease Center, which was renamed in 1970 when its functions were broadened to include, in addition to its traditional activities related to infectious disease, other preventable conditions including malnutrition.

[23]February 1974.

Table 4–4. Department of Health, Education and Welfare, 1974. [a]

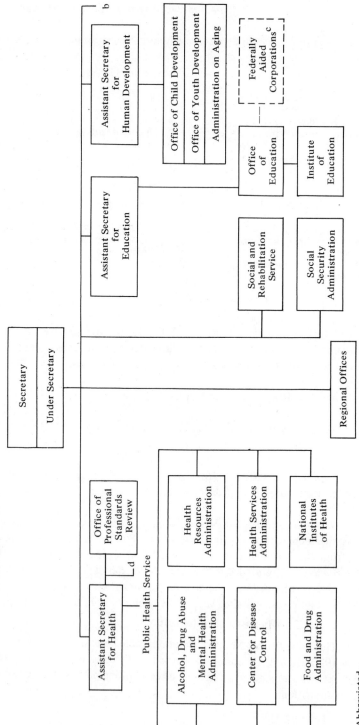

[a] Abbreviated

[b] Also Assistant Secretaries for Public Affairs, Legislation Planning and Evaluation, Administration and Management

[c] American Printing House for the Blind, Gallaudet College, Howard University

[d] Also: Office of International Health, Office of Population Affairs, Office of Drug Abuse Prevention, Office of Nursing Home Affairs.

The Center conducts and supports programs for prevention and control of disease and administers the National Clearinghouse for Smoking and Health. It provides consultation and assistance to state and local health departments and other countries, including extensive epidemiological services. It is also responsible for foreign quarantine activities.

Under the 1973 Public Health Service reorganization, the Center incorporated the National Institute of Occupational Safety and Health,[24] including the Appalachian Laboratory of Occupational Respiratory Disease. It also took over from the former Bureau of Community Environmental Management the functions related to lead poisoning prevention and rat control.

Food and Drug Administration. This agency is responsible for determining the safety of foods, drugs, cosmetics, and therapeutic devices; for proper labeling and product information; and approval of all new drugs for marketing. The 1962 Kefauver-Harris amendments to the Pure Food, Drug and Cosmetics Act require in addition that the FDA consider efficacy as well as safety in making decisions regarding drugs and therapeutic devices.

Health Resources Administration

National Center for Health Statistics. The Center collects and reports the official U.S. vital statistics. It carries out a continuing program of studies, data evaluation and methods research in health and vital statistics. These include special continuing surveys, including:

1. The *Health Interview Survey*—a national household interview study of illness, disability, and health services utilization.[25]
2. The *Health Examination Survey*—a program of examination and testing of national population samples.
3. The *Master Facility Inventory Survey*—periodically surveys all U.S. health facilities.
4. The *Ambulatory Medical Care Survey* was begun in 1973. Data is collected from a sample of practicing physicians.

Bureau of Health Services Research

Conducts and supports research and demonstration projects related to the financing, organization and delivery of health care. Special emphasis has been given to the areas of cost, quality and new types of health manpower. (As of this writing, the organization of the Bureau is in process.)

---

[24] The National Institute of Occupational Safety and Health conducts research and studies and develops standards in this area.

[25] This was the first system for the regular collection of health related data by the Public Health Service. It was developed under the National Health Survey Act of 1956.

Bureau of Health Resources Development

1. *Comprehensive Health Planning Service.* Administers the comprehensive health planning grants program under the Comprehensive Health Planning legislation. This includes support for state and area health planning agencies and for manpower development in health planning.
2. *Health Care Facilities Service.* Administers the Hill-Burton program of grants, loans, and consultation for the construction and modernization of health facilities.
3. *Regional Medical Programs Service.* Administers the Regional Medical Programs.[26]

The health manpower development activities of the Public Health Service, including grant support for education and training, are consolidated in the Bureau in the following divisions:

Division of Physician and Health Professions Education
Division of Nursing
Division of Dental Health
Division of Allied Health Manpower
Division of Manpower Intelligence

Health Services Administration

Indian Health Service. This agency administers the system of hospitals and health centers which provides health services to American Indians and native Alaskans.

Federal Health Programs Service. This service administers the Public Health Service[27] hospitals and clinics, and provides work related health services for federal employees. Its Division of Emergency Health Services supports emergency medical care training programs and provides medical assistance in disasters.

Bureau of Community Health Services. This agency administers programs related to maternal and child health,[28] family planning, comprehensive

---

[26]Termination of these programs is anticipated.

[27]Eight general hospitals and a hospital for leprosy patients in Carvill, Louisiana. (In 1948, there were 24 hospitals. Many have since been closed or turned over to local communities.)

[28]Maternal and Child Health and Crippled Children's Services (Title V of the Social Security Act).

health centers (neighborhood health centers), migrant health, and health maintenance organization development. It also includes the *National Health Service Corps,* a program for deployment of Public Health Service personnel, including physicians, to areas of particular need.

Bureau of Quality Assurance. This agency promotes and supports activities related to standards and evaluation. It cooperates with state agencies in activities related to standards for services under Medicare and Medicaid and other federal health care programs.

National Institutes of Health. This agency, nominally with the Public Health Service, includes the National Library of Medicine,[29] the Fogarty International Center for the Advanced Study of Health Sciences, and ten *research institutes:*

National Cancer Institute
National Heart and Lung Institute
National Institute of Dental Research
National Institute of Neurological Disease and Stroke[30]
National Institute of Arthritis, Metabolism and Digestive Diseases[31]
National Institute of Allergy and Infectious Diseases
National Institute of Child Health and Human Development
National Institute of General Medical Sciences
National Eye Institute
National Institute of Environmental Health Sciences

The National Institutes carry out and support programs of basic and clinical research.

Social Security Administration
The Social Security Administration is responsible for the Old Age, Survivors, and Disability Insurance Program (OASDI) and for administering most of the program of Health Insurance for the Aged (Medicare). It administers the recently established program of Supplemental Security Income for the Aged, Blind and Disabled.[32] It is also responsible for review and authorization of claims for black-lung benefits under the Federal Coal Mine Health and Safety Act of

---

[29]The Library carries on a wide variety of informational activities, including publication of the *Index Medicus,* and development and operation of the Medical Literature and Analysis Retrieval System (MEDLARS).

[30]Originally the National Institute of Neurological Disease and Blindness.

[31]Previously the National Institute of Arthritis and Metabolic Disease.

[32]Effective January 1974, under provisions of the Social Security Amendments of 1972.

1969. The *Office of Research and Statistics* collects and analyzes data concerning health costs and expenditures and publishes many reports.

The divisions of the Social Security Administration are:

Bureau of Data Processing
Bureau of Disability Insurance
Bureau of District Office Operations
Bureau of Health Insurance
Bureau of Hearings and Appeals
Bureau of Retirement and Survivors Insurance
Bureau of Supplemental Security Income for the Aged, Blind, and Disabled

Social and Rehabilitation Service

The Social and Rehabilitation Service administers programs of grants-in-aid to the states for:

1. Public assistance to families with dependent children (Aid to Families with Dependent Children, AFDC).
2. Medical assistance (Medicaid).
3. Social services under the AFDC program including foster care, day care, and family planning services.
4. Social services for aged, blind, and disabled adults.
5. Vocational rehabilitation of the disabled.
6. Services and facilities for persons with developmental disabilities, including mental retardation.[33]

The divisions of the Social and Rehabilitation Service are:

Assistance Payments Administration
Community Services Administration
Medical Services Administration
Rehabilitation Services Administration

Division of Education

Office of Education. The Office of Education has retained its original statutory mandate to gather statistics and diffuse information concerning education. In addition, it administers many grant programs related to elementary, secondary, and higher education. The Office also sets standards and criteria for the recognition, for purposes of federal funding, of voluntary agencies which accredit educational institutions and programs (including those engaged in *health manpower education* and training).

---

[33]Under the Developmental Disabilities Services and Facilities Construction Act.

National Institute of Education. The Institute of Education was established in 1972 to coordinate research and development programs in education.

Regional Offices
There are ten regional offices[34] of the Department of Health, Education and Welfare, where the operating agencies maintain staffs who work cooperatively with state and local government and community agencies in carrying out departmental programs. Their responsibilities include the review and approval of grant applications.

References
United States Government Manual, official handbook of the Federal Government, published annually by the office of the Federal Register (General Services Administration).

Annual reports of the Department of Health, Education and Welfare, U.S. Government Printing Office, 1953-1971.

3. INTRODUCTION TO HEALTH LEGISLATION

The many activities of the federal government in health are authorized by the passage of laws, or statutes, by the Congress.

The Enactment of Laws[35]

Proposed legislation, called a *bill,*[36] is introduced in the Senate or House of Representatives by a congressional sponsor.[37] It is assigned a sequential number (i.e., HR-1, S-3) and referred to the appropriate committee for study. Public *hearings* are often held, after which the bill may be amended or entirely redrafted, sometimes in combination with other bills addressed to the same issue. Ultimately, if it is approved, the bill is discharged from the committee with a favorable report and is then placed on the legislative calendar for floor action. (A committee does not act on every bill referred to it and there is no time limit within which it must report out a bill.)

If passed by the Senate or House (with or without amendments from the floor), the bill is sent to the other chamber where essentially the same process of committee referral, reporting, and floor debate takes place.

---

[34]The offices are: I Boston, II New York, III Philadelphia, IV Atlanta, V Chicago, VI Dallas, VII Kansas City, Mo., VIII Denver, IX San Francisco, X Seattle.

[35]This is a general outline of a very complex process.

[36]Some legislation is introduced as *resolutions,* which have essentially the same practical significance as bills.

[37]Legislation may be drafted by legislators and their staffs, by various levels of the Executive Branch, or by private citizens or groups. A bill may have a number of Congressional sponsors, up to 25 in the House and unlimited in the Senate.

If there is substantial disagreement between the two houses on a bill which has been passed by both, *Conference Committees* will be formed from among the members of the committees which reported the bill. If an agreement is arrived at, a *conference report* is made which is then voted on as a whole, without amendment, by each house. If passed by both houses it is sent to the President for approval. When signed by him, the bill becomes a law or *statute.*

Any legislation which has not been finally passed by both the Senate and House of Representatives by the end of a Congress[38] is dead and must be re-introduced in the next Congress if it is to be again considered. (Only a minority of the many bills introduced in each legislative session become a law.)

The law is then numbered sequentially and by number of the Congress; for example, Public Law 89-97 (PL 89-97) means the 97th law passed by the 89th Congress.[39] The law is printed in pamphlet form known as a *slip law;* later it is published in the *Statutes at Large* and ultimately incorporated into the *United States Code.*

The formal title, which is an integral part of the law, takes the form "An Act to . . ." and may be quite detailed. Often a *short title* is also specified. Frequently, however, a law comes to be known by the names of its chief Congressional sponsors.

For example, PL79-725 is formally entitled "An Act to amend the Public Health Service Act to authorize grants to the states for surveying their hospital and public health centers and for planning construction of additional facilities, and to authorize grants to assist in such construction." Its short title is the "Hospital Survey and Construction Act." However, it is generally known as the "Hill-Burton Act" after its sponsors, Senators Lister Hill and Harold Burton.

Rarely, a law will retain as its popular name its original bill number, notably the Social Security Amendments of 1972, which are still widely referred to as "HR-1."

Occasionally a specific section of an Act may be given a specific short title. For example, Title (section) I of PL 92-157 is the Comprehensive Health Manpower Training Act of 1971.

Sometimes a part of a law will acquire a popular name. For example, the Professional Standards Review Organizations (PSRO) section of the Social Security Amendments of 1972 is often called the "Bennett Amendment" after Senator Wallace Bennett, who amended the original bill with these provisions.

Much legislation is "authorizing" legislation which establishes or continues programs and authorizes funding for them. *Appropriations bills* actually provide the funds. Often, less is appropriated than has been

---

[38]The two annual sessions spanning the term of office of members of the House of Representatives are known as a Congress. For example, the 92nd Congress extended from January 1971 to December 1972.

[39]There is also a series of *Private Laws* relating to private individuals or claims against the government.

authorized to be appropriated. Furthermore, the Executive branch may not elect to spend all the funds appropriated for a particular purpose if these were more than requested or if it does not wish to implement a particular program.

The actual power of the President to "impound" funds appropriated by the Congress is a Constitutional question which remains unsettled and which has been a focus of controversy between the Executive and Legislative branches of the government.

Many of the details of the various laws are left to be spelled out in *regulations* prescribed by the various administrative agencies of the Executive Branch. As these are made, they are published in the *Federal Register,* taking effect 30 days thereafter. These regulations are then incorporated in the *Code of Federal Regulations* and have the force of law.

Congressional Committees

There are 17 standing committees in the Senate and 21 in the House of Representatives. Many committees may be involved in the various matters relating to health, but those of particular importance are:

House Ways and Means Committee[40]
Senate Finance Committee: Subcommittee on Health
House Interstate and Foreign Commerce Committee: Subcommittee on Public Health and Environment
Senate Labor and Public Welfare Committee: Subcommittee on Health
House Appropriations Committee: Subcommittee for Labor and Health, Education, and Welfare
Senate Appropriations Committee: Subcommittee for Labor and Health, Education and Welfare

Grants-in-Aid

Many of the funds distributed to the states and localities under federal legislation are made available by the mechanism of *grants-in-aid.* These grants are authorized in the various federal laws for stated purposes and are given to the states and to local organizations, agencies and individuals, under certain conditions and in accordance with certain regulations.

Formula grants—Funds are allotted by a formula which takes into consideration such factors as state population, per capita income, and the extent of health problems.

Matching grants—Funds must be matched up to a specified percentage by the state, agency, or institution receiving the grant. For example, for construction grants under Hill-Burton program: "The Federal share shall be . . . not more than 66 2/3 percent."

---

[40]Has jurisdiction over the Social Security laws, due to the Constitutional provision that laws to raise revenue must originate in the House; such (tax) measures are assigned to this committee.

Research grants—Funds are granted competitively to individuals, agencies, and institutions to carry out specific research work outlined in research proposals submitted by the applicants.

Training grants—Funds are granted competitively to institutions engaged in certain health manpower training activities. These may include student stipends.

Capitation grants—Funds are allotted to educational institutions by formulas related to student enrollment.

"Categorical grants" are made for relatively narrowly defined categories of problems, i.e., entities such as chronic disease, venereal disease.

"Block grants" are for more broadly defined purposes, such as public health services in general, and permit more discretion in use of the funds.

Grants-in-aid to the states are usually made from allotments among the states in accordance with the specified formula. These grants also carry such requirements as the submission of a *state plan* concerning the problem or purpose in question, assignment of the responsibility for administration of the plan to a *single state agency* and conformation to guidelines and standards regarding use of the funds. They are typically formula grants, and generally have matching requirements.

Programs of grants-in-aid are usually authorized for stipulated periods of time only, usually two to five years; these authorizations must be renewed periodically if programs are to continue. Thus, at any point in time, several of these will be in various stages of the legislative process, for continuation and amendment.[41]

The concept of *revenue sharing* has been advocated as a more appropriate mechanism for financial aid to the states than the relatively categorical approach of the grant-in-aid programs. The first revenue sharing legislation was passed in 1972.[42] Whether such a mechanism should ultimately largely replace the grant-in-aid structure, especially in the health field, has been a subject of some controversy.

Specific Health Legislation

The following sections summarize the principal federal legislation related to health care. They do not attempt to deal with the complex political, social, and economic background of this body of legislation, nor with its implementation and impact. They are designed to provide a base from which to address these issues.

---

[41] One exception is the research and training grants of The National Institutes of Health which have no statutory time limit, though subject to the usual appropriations bills.

[42] The State and Local Fiscal Assistance Act of 1972. Funds are allocated to state governments with relatively few restrictions. Local governments must use their funds for "priority expenditures": necessary capital expenditures, and operating expenses in the areas of public safety, environmental protection, public transportation, health, recreation, libraries, social service for the poor and aged, and financial administration.

The material is presented in such a way as to give a general sense of the historical development of these laws which have had and will continue to have a profound effect on the health care scene.

The Social Security Act, and the Public Health Service Act are described in particular detail, as they have been the vehicles for such important health-related programs as Medicare, Medicaid, Hill-Burton and Comprehensive Health Planning.

References

Robert H. Hamlin, *Public Health Law or the Interrelationships of Law and Public Health Administration, American Journal of Public Health* 51:1733, 1961. A good review of some basic concepts and terminology.

Floyd M. Riddick, *Enactment of a Law* Senate Document 35, 1967.

Charles I. Zinn, *How Our Laws Are Made,* House of Representatives Document 125, 1969.

Guide to the Congress (Washington D.C.: Congressional Quarterly, 1971).

The Department of Health, Education and Welfare: Background Material Concerning the Mission and Organization of the Health Activities of the Department, prepared for the Special subcommittee on HEW Investigation, Interstate and Foreign Commerce Committee, (U.S. Government Printing Office, 1966). Section VII, Grants-in-aid, pp. 113-262 is a detailed description of the grant-in-aid programs of the Public Health Service as of 1966, illustrating the scope and complexity of the programs.

NOTE: There are many official *government document depositories,* containing selected documents, in public and university libraries throughout the country. Some of these are *regional depositories* which receive copies of most documents published by the Government Printing Office.

4. THE SOCIAL SECURITY ACT

An Act to provide for the federal welfare by establishing a system of federal old age benefits, and by enabling the several States to make more adequate provision for aged persons, blind persons, dependent and crippled children, maternal and child welfare, public health, and the administration of their unemployment compensation laws; to establish a Social Security Board: to raise revenue; and for other purposes.

The Social Security Act of 1935 was a landmark piece of legislation which was developed and passed during the Great Depression. It represented the first major entrance of the federal government into the area of social insurance and it greatly and significantly expanded federal grant-in-aid assistance to the states. It has formed the base for important federal programs in health including, most recently, Medicare and Medicaid.

The original legislation consisted of eleven Titles (divisions):

Title I. Grants to the States for Old Age Assistance
Provided grants to the states for financial assistance to needy aged.

Title II. Federal Old Age Benefits
Set up the federal "Social Security" program of old age benefits based on wages earned before age 65.[43]

Title III. Grants to the States for Unemployment Compensation Administration
Provided federal payment for the administrative expenses of state programs for unemployment compensation.

Title IV. Grants to the States for Aid to Dependent Children
Provided for grants to the states for financial aid for needy dependent children.[44]

Title V. Grants to the States for Maternal and Child Welfare
Provided grants to the states for maternal and child health and child welfare services, and services to crippled children. Administration of the program was assigned to the Children's Bureau.[45] (Also extended vocational rehabilitation programs previously authorized under other legislation.)

Title VI. Public Health Work
Provided grants to the states for state and local public health services and additional funds for programs of the Public Health Service.

Title VII. Social Security Board
Established the Social Security Board to administer the programs authorized under the Act (with the exception of those in Titles V and VI), and to study and make recommendations regarding economic security and social insurance.

Title VIII. Taxes with Respect to Employment
Levied a payroll tax on employees eligible for the federal old age benefits program, and a tax in equal amount on their employers.

Title IX. Tax on Employers of Eight or More
Levied an additional tax on employers which could be credited against contributions to state unemployment funds. Its purpose was to encourage the establishment of such funds by the states.

---

[43] There were many exclusions in the original Act, including domestic and agricultural labor, employees of governmental and non-profit agencies, and the self-employed. Coverage since has been gradually extended and at present includes more than 90 percent of working people. (Railway workers are similarly covered under the Railroad Retirement Act; federal employees also have a separate program.)

[44] Children under age 16 deprived of parental support through death, absence or incapacity of a parent, and living with relatives. Payments are now authorized for children up to age 21 providing they are in school.

[45] This Title in effect re-established and expanded the program of assistance for maternal and child health programs previously authorized under the federal Maternity and Infancy Act (1921–29) which was the first federal grant-in-aid program for direct health services.

Title X.   *Grants to the States for Aid to the Blind*
Provided grants to the states for financial assistance to needy blind persons.
Title XI.   *General Provisions*
Contained general definitions and administrative regulations.

In summary, the Act:

1. Established the "Social Security" program of old age benefits.
2. Provided for federal financial assistance to the states' public assistance ("welfare") programs.
3. Provided fiscal incentives for the establishment of state unemployment funds.
4. Greatly increased financial assistance to the states for state and local public health programs and established such assistance for maternal and child health and child welfare services.

Amendments

In the ensuing years there have been many amendments of the original Social Security Act. Especially noteworthy are the following:

1939—Benefits for *dependents* and *survivors* were added to the old age program. The program was now known as Old Age and Survivors Insurance (OASI).
1950—The program of federal aid to state public assistance programs was extended to *disabled persons* (Title XIV). Federal participation in state payments to providers of medical services (*vendor payments*) to persons on public assistance was also added.
1956—A federal program of disability benefits was added to OASI. The program was now known as Old Age, Survivors and Disability Insurance (OASDI).
1960—The Kerr-Mills Act established a program of *medical assistance* to the needy aged, providing payments for medical care for needy elderly persons not receiving public assistance ("medically indigent aged"). This was the forerunner of the Medicaid program.
1963—The Maternal and Child Health and Mental Retardation Planning Amendments included the authorization of special project grants for comprehensive programs of maternity care for women in low income families and for their infants.
1965—Two new sections were added: Health Insurance for the Aged (Title XVIII, *Medicare*) and Grants to the States for Medical Assistance Programs (Title XIX, *Medicaid*); and special project grants for *children and youth* programs were authorized.
1967—A number of adjustments were made in the Medicare and Medicaid programs including provision for limitation of federal participation in the latter.

1972—Many amendments were made to the Medicare and Medicaid programs, including the inclusion of persons receiving federal disability benefits in Medicare and the establishment of Professional Standards Review Organizations (PSRO); a new federal minimum income program, Supplemental Security Income, (under a new Title XVI) replaced the federally aided adult public assistance programs.[46]

The 1960 and subsequent amendments are described in some detail in the following pages.

5.   SOCIAL SECURITY AMENDMENTS OF 1960
"KERR-MILLS ACT"

The 1960 Social Security Amendments made a number of changes and extensions of various titles of the Act. The most important provisions were those related to medical services for the aged, provisions which were passed after extensive congressional debate concerning health insurance for the aged.

Medical Assistance for the Aged

Title I of the Social Security Act was amended to read *Grants to the States for Old Age Assistance and Medical Assistance for the Aged:*

> . . . for the purpose of enabling each state to furnish medical assistance on behalf of aged individuals who are not recipients of old age assistance but whose income and resources are insufficient to meet the costs of necessary medical services . . .

This established a new program of *medical assistance for the aged* (MAA) providing for federal aid to the states for payments for medical care for "medically indigent" persons age 65 and over. This became known as the Kerr-Mills program.

Participation by the states was optional. Under the program:

1. A broad range of medical services could be made available with the stipulation that at least *some institutional* and *some non-institutional* care be available to the recipients.
2. No lien could be made on a recipient's property during his lifetime (and lifetime of spouse).

---

[46] "Federally Aided Public Assistance Categories"

State welfare programs which were eligible for federal assistance were those directed to the elderly, to families with dependent children, to the blind and the disabled. The federal assistance categories were:

1. Old Age Assistance (OAA)
2. Aid to Families with Dependent Children
3. Aid to the Blind (AB)
4. Aid to the Permanently and Totally Disabled (APTD)

3. No duration of residence requirement could be made for any person residing in the state.
4. Federal participation to be 50-80 percent of program costs, according to per capita income in the state.
5. Federal sharing was excluded for payments for persons in non-medical institutions and persons in tuberculosis and mental hospitals.

Additionally, increased federal funding was provided for medical services under the existing state old age assistance (OAA) programs.

6. MATERNAL AND CHILD HEALTH AND MENTAL RETARDATION PLANNING AMENDMENTS OF 1963

An Act to amend the Social Security Act to assist States and communities in preventing and combating mental retardation through expansion and improvement of the maternal and child health and crippled children's programs, through provision of prenatal, maternity, and infant care for individuals with conditions associated with childbearing which may lead to mental retardation, and through planning for comprehensive action to combat mental retardation, and for other purposes.

The 1963 Social Security Amendments made several additions to Title V:

1. Increased funds were authorized for Maternal and Child Health and Crippled Children's Services
2. Special Project Grants for Maternity and Infant Care—"In order to help reduce the incidence of mental retardation caused by complications associated with childbearing" there were authorized to state health agencies and, with the consent of such agency, to any local health agency grants for "projects for the provision of necessary health care to prospective mothers (including, after childbirth, health care to mothers and their infants) who have or are likely to have conditions associated with childbearing which increase the hazards to the health of the mothers or their infants . . . and whom the state or local health agency determines will not receive necessary health care because they are from low income families or for other reasons beyond their control." Federal participation: 75 percent of costs.
3. Grants were also authorized for *research projects* relating to maternal and child health services and crippled children's services.

A new title was also added to the Social Security Act: Title XVII, *Grants for Planning Comprehensive Action to Combat Mental Retardation.*

Grants were authorized to assist the states to plan for comprehensive state and community action to combat mental retardation.[47] Federal participation: 75 percent of costs.

7. SOCIAL SECURITY AMENDMENTS OF 1965 *

An Act to provide a hospital insurance program for the aged under the Social Security Act with a supplementary medical benefits program and an expanded program of medical assistance, to increase benefits under the Old-Age, Survivors, and Disability Insurance System, to improve the Federal-State public assistance programs, and for other purposes.

The Social Security amendments of 1965 established the national program of health insurance for the aged now known as "Medicare."[48] It was the culmination of many years of national and Congressional debate and is of great historic importance. The amendments also included provisions for expansion of the Kerr-Mills medical assistance program to groups other than the elderly—a program now known as "Medicaid." Significant additions were made to Title V, and changes were also made in the OASDI and Public Assistance titles of the Social Security Act.

Health Insurance for the Aged (Medicare)

Title XVIII, *Health Insurance for the Aged,* was added to the Social Security Act. Because of the importance of this legislation, a relatively extensive summary of the original provisions is set forth below.

Part A: Hospital Insurance Benefits. This insurance program provides basic protection against the costs of hospital and related post-hospital services. Benefits consist of entitlement to have payment made for:

1. *Inpatient hospital* services up to 90 days during any spell of illness and psychiatric inpatient services up to 190 days lifetime.
2. Post-hospital *extended care* services up to 100 days during any spell of illness.
3. Post-hospital *home health* services up to 100 visits in a one-year period.
4. Hospital outpatient *diagnostic* services.

---

[47]*PL 89-97. This provision for planning grants has since expired.

[48]This term was originally applied to the program for medical care for servicemen's dependents under the Dependents Medical Care Act (1956). It is now universally applied to this program of health insurance for the aged.

handwritten margin note: medicaid; title XIX "grants to the states for medical assistance programs," was added to the social security act.

The amount payable for these services (except home health) is subject to deductible and coinsurance payments by the beneficiary as follows:[49]

1. *Inpatient:* $40 deductible until January 1, 1969, thereafter to be increased according to the increase in average per diem rates for in-hospital services;[50] coinsurance, equal to one-fourth the deductible, for each day after the sixtieth hospital day.
2. *Extended care:* no deductible; coinsurance, equal to one-eight the inpatient hospital deductible, for each day after the twentieth day.
3. *Home health services:* no deductible or coinsurance.
4. *Outpatient:* for services provided in a 20-day period by one hospital, deductible is equal to one-half the inpatient deductible; coinsurance is equal to 20 percent of the remaining amount payable.

The *conditions for payment to providers* of service include:

1. Written request by beneficiary (except where found impracticable by the Secretary).
2. *Certification* by a physician of the necessity for the services, and periodic recertification where applicable, beginning no later than the twentieth day.
3. For psychiatric hospital services, certification that such treatment can reasonably be expected to *improve the condition* for which treatment is necessary.
4. For tuberculosis hospital services, certification that treatment can reasonably be expected to *improve the condition* or render it non-communicable.
5. For post-hospital extended care services, certification of the need for *skilled nursing care* for condition for which the preceding inpatient services were received.
6. For post-hospital home health services, certification that services are required because the individual is confined to his home and needs *skilled nursing care,* or physical or speech therapy for conditions for which he was receiving inpatient hospital services.

The amount paid to any provider of services must be the *reasonable cost* of such services.

Payment may be made for emergency services provided by a nonparticipating hospital including, under limited conditions, hospitals outside the United States.

---

[49] See pp. 81-82 for discussion of deductibles and coinsurance.

[50] The deductible was considered to represent roughly the cost of the first hospital day.

Groups of associations of providers of services may elect to have payments made through a public or private agency or organization.[51] The Secretary is authorized to make agreements with such designated organizations by which they will determine the payments to be made for services and will make such payments. These agencies may be required to:

1. Provide consultation to providers for their establishment of necessary fiscal records and the meeting of other qualifications.
2. Serve as a center for communication of information between the Secretary and the providers.
3. Make necessary audits of records of providers.

The nomination of an agency or organization, however, is not binding on individual members of the nominating association or group.

A *Federal Hospital Insurance Trust Fund* is established for payments under Part A. The trust fund is to be financed by an earnings tax paid by employees, employers and the self-employed.

Part B: Supplementary Medical Insurance Benefits. This is a voluntary insurance program financed from premium payments by enrollees and contributions from federal funds. Benefits consist of entitlement to have payment made for:

1. Home health services up to 100 visits in a year.
2. Medical and other health services:
   a. *physicians'* services
   b. *services and supplies* incident to a physician's professional services
   c. *diagnostic X-ray,* laboratory, and other tests
   d. *radio-therapy*
   e. *surgical dressings,* splints, casts
   f. *rental of durable medical equipment* used in the home
   g. *ambulance service* (with limitations)
   h. *prosthetic devices* (except dental) and *braces*

Independent laboratories providing services under this program must be approved by the Secretary.

Payments for *physicians' services* are to be 80 percent of *reasonable charges,* and may be made to the beneficiary or on his behalf. (An organization providing services on a prepayment basis may be paid 80 percent of reasonable costs.)

---

[51]These non-federal agencies which deal directly with the providers of services are known as *fiscal intermediaries.*

Payments for other medical and health services are to be 80 percent of *reasonable costs.*

Medical and other health services under this part are subject to a $50 deductible in each calendar year. (Expenses incurred for hospital outpatient diagnostic services under Part A may be counted toward the deductible.)

With regard to out of hospital *psychiatric services,* there shall be considered as incurred expense in any year, no more than $250 after the deductible.

The *conditions for payment to providers* of services include:

1. Written *request by beneficiary,* unless impracticable.
2. In the case of *home health* services, *certification by a physician* that the individual is confined to his home and needs skilled nursing care or physical or speech therapy and that services are furnished while the individual is *under the care of a physician.*
3. In the case of other medical or health services, certification by a physician, that these were *medically required.*

Provision is made for general and individual *enrollment periods.*

The *initial monthly premium is set at $3.* Beginning in 1968, the monthly premium shall be determined every two years on the basis of the benefit and administrative costs of the program.

For persons receiving monthly Social Security benefits, premiums will be deducted from these payments.

A *Federal Supplementary Insurance Trust Fund* is established for payments under Part B.

The Surgeon General is authorized to enter into *contracts with (health insurance) carriers* for administration of these benefits. The carriers will:

1. Determine rates and amounts of payments required, disburse and account for funds, and make necessary audits of records of providers of services.
2. Assist in development of procedures relating to utilization practices and determine compliance with requirements for utilization review.
3. Serve as a channel for communication of information relating to the administration of this program.
4. Assure that payments are made for reasonable costs, and for charges which are reasonable and not higher than the charges applicable for comparable services to the policyholders and subscribers of the carrier. Payments for charges may be made on the basis of a receipted bill or on the basis of an *assignment.* In the latter case the reasonable charge will be the full charge for the services.

In determining the reasonable charge for services there shall be taken into consideration the *customary charges* for similar services generally made by physicians or other persons furnishing such services, as well as the *prevailing* charges in the locality.

The Surgeon General, at the request of a state, will enter into an agreement whereby eligible individuals in the federally aided *public assistance categories* will be enrolled in Part B with the monthly premium to be paid by the state.

A government contribution will be made from the Treasury *equal to the aggregate premiums* payable under this part.[52]

Part C: Miscellaneous Provisions. Definitions[53] (for purposes of Title XVIII) include:

1. Spell of Illness—a period beginning with the first day on which an individual is furnished inpatient hospital services or extended care services and ending with the close of the first period of 60 consecutive days thereafter on each of which he is neither an inpatient of a hospital or an extended care facility.
2. Inpatient Hospital Service
   a. Bed and board.
   b. Such nursing services, use of hospital facilities, medical social services, and such drugs, biological supplies, appliances, and equipment, for use in the hospital, as are ordinarily furnished to in-patients by a hospital. *Excluded* are *physicians'* services (except interns and residents under a training program) and the services of *private duty nurses.*
3. Hospital—an institution which:
   a. Is primarily engaged in providing by or under the supervision of physicians, to in-patients, services for diagnosis, treatment, care, or rehabilitation.
   b. Maintains clinical records on all patients.
   c. Has bylaws in effect with respect to its staff of physicians.
   d. Has a requirement that every patient must be under the care of a physician.
   e. Provides *24-hour nursing service* rendered or supervised by a registered professional nurse.
   f. Has in effect a hospital *utilization review plan.*
   g. If in any state whose laws provide for licensing of hospitals, is so licensed or meets the standards for licensure.
   h. Meets such other requirements as the Secretary finds necessary in the interest of the health and safety of hospitalized individuals except that such requirements may not be higher than the comparable requirements of the Joint Commission on Accreditation of Hospitals.

---

[52] i.e., half the costs of Part B will be paid from general revenues.
[53] Abbreviated.

4. Extended Care Facility[54]—an institution (or distinct part of an institution) which has in effect a *transfer agreement* with one or more participating hospitals and which:

   a. Is primarily engaged in providing to inpatients *skilled nursing care* or *rehabilitation* services.

   b. Has policies which are developed with the advice of a group of professional personnel, and has a physician, a registered professional nurse or a medical staff responsible for the execution of such policies.

   c. Requires that every patient be under the supervision of a physician and provides for having a physician available in case of emergency.

   d. Maintains clinical records on all patients.

   e. Provides *24-hour nursing service* sufficient to meet nursing needs in accordance with the policies developed and has *at least one registered nurse employed full time.*

   f. Provides appropriate methods and procedures for the dispensing and administering of drugs and biologicals.

   g. Has a *utilization review plan.*

   h. If in any state with laws providing for licensing of such institutions, is so *licensed* or meets the licensure standards.

   i. Meets such other conditions relating to the health and safety of its patients as the Secretary may find necessary.

5. Utilization Review—a utilization review plan of a hospital or extended care facility is considered sufficient if it is applicable to services to individuals entitled to insurance benefits under this title. It is to provide:

   a. For a review, on a sample or other basis, of admissions, *duration of stay* and professional services with respect to *medical necessity* and to promote the most efficient use of facilities and services.

   b. For review to be made by a staff committee of *two or more physicians,* with or without other professional personnel or a similar group established by the local medical society and some or all of the hospitals and extended care facilities in the locality.

   c. For review of cases of *extended duration.*

   d. For prompt notification to the institution, the individual, and his physician of any finding (made after opportunity for consultation with such physician) that further stay in the institution is not medically necessary.

6. Home Health Agency—an agency or organization which:

   a. Is primarily engaged in providing skilled nursing services and other therapeutic services.

   b. *Has policies established by a group of professional personnel* including one or more physicians and one or more registered professional nurses,

---

[54]This term has since been superseded by the term *Skilled Nursing Facility.*

and provides for supervision of such services by a physician or a registered professional nurse.

c. Maintains clinical records on all patients.

d. If in any state providing for the licensing of organizations of this nature, is so *licensed* or meets the licensure standards.

e. Meets *such other conditions of participation* as the Secretary may find necessary in the interest of individuals furnished services.

7. Home Health Services—the following items and services furnished to an individual under the care of a physician by a home health agency on a visiting basis in an individual's home:

   a. Nursing care provided by or under the supervision of a registered professional nurse.

   b. *Physical, occupational,* or *speech* therapy.

   c. Medical *social services.*

   d. *Home health aid* services.

   e. Medical *supplies* and use of medical *appliances.*

   f. Any of the foregoing provided on an outpatient basis at a hospital, extended care facility, or rehabilitation center which involves the use of equipment which cannot be made readily available in the home.

8. Post-Hospital Extended Care Services—extended care service furnished an individual after transfer from a hospital in which he was an inpatient for not less than *3 consecutive days;* admission to the extended care facility to be not more than *14 days* after discharge from such hospital.

9. Post-Hospital Home Health Services—home health services furnished an individual within one year after his most recent discharge from a hospital of which he was an inpatient for not less than *3 consecutive days,* or from an extended care facility (in which he was an inpatient under Part A). In either case, the plan for home health services is to be established *within 14 days* after such discharge.

10. Physician—a licensed doctor of medicine, osteopathy, or dentistry.

11. Provider of Services—a hospital, extended care facility, or home health agency.

Payment is to be made for the reasonable cost of *semi-private* accommodations: two-bed, three-bed, or four-bed. Payment may exceed semi-private cost only if more expensive accommodations are required for medical reasons. If accommodations furnished are less expensive than semi-private, payment will be minus the difference.

Excluded from coverage are (among others):

1. Services which are not provided within the United States (except emergency services).

2. Personal comfort items.

3. Routine physical *checkups*; *eyeglasses* or related eye examinations; *hearing aids* or related examinations; *immunizations.*
4. *Orthopedic* shoes or other supportive devices for the feet.
5. *Custodial care.*
6. Cosmetic surgery except as required for repair of accidental injury or improvement of functioning of a malformed body member.
7. Care, treatment, filling, removal, or replacement of teeth.
8. Services provided under a workmen's compensation law.

In developing *conditions of participation for providers of services* the Secretary shall consult with the Health Insurance Benefits Advisory Council, appropriate state agencies, recognized national listing or accrediting bodies and may consult with appropriate local agencies.

The Secretary shall make an agreement with any state willing and able to do so whereby an appropriate state or local agency may determine whether an institution is a hospital or extended care facility, or an agency is a home health agency (as these terms are defined) or whether a laboratory meets the stated requirements. The Secretary may also agree to utilize the services of such agencies to:

> Provide consultation to institutions or agencies to assist them to establish and maintain fiscal records or otherwise to qualify as providers of services, including the establishment of utilization review procedures.

The requirements for a participating hospital shall be deemed to have been met if an institution is accredited as a hospital by the *Joint Commission on Accreditation of Hospitals* (provided that utilization review procedures are also established).[55]

A *Health Insurance Benefits Advisory Council* of 16 members is established to advise the Secretary on general policy in the administration of this Title and in the formulation of regulations. Members to include persons in fields related to hospital, medical and other health activities and at least one person representing the general public.

A *National Medical Review Committee* of 9 members is established to include individuals who are representative of organizations and associations of professional personnel in the field of medicine, other individuals from medicine or related fields, and at least one member representative of the general public; a majority of the members to be physicians. The function of the Committee is to study the utilization of hospital and other medical care and services provided under this Title with a view to *recommending any changes* which may seem

---

[55] Accreditation by the American Osteopathic Association or other national accreditation body may also be accepted.

desirable *in the way in which such services are utilized* and in the *administration of the programs* established by this Title.

The Secretary shall *prescribe such regulations* as may be necessary to carry out the administration of this program.

Eligibility. Persons eligible are those who have attained the age of 65 and are entitled to monthly social security or railroad retirement benefits. Other persons are eligible under transitional provisions, provided they attain age 65 before 1968 and are resident citizens of the United States or have been permanent resident aliens for at least five years. Excluded are those eligible for the Federal Employee Health Benefits Program and those convicted of specific crimes against national security.

Grants to the States for Medical Assistance (Medicaid)

Title XIX, *Grants to the States for Medical Assistance Programs,* was added to the Social Security Act:

> For the purpose of enabling each state to furnish medical assistance on behalf of families with dependent children and of aged, blind, or permanently and totally disabled individuals whose income and resources are insufficient to meet the costs of necessary medical services. . . .

This Title establishes a single *new program of medical assistance* for persons receiving federally aided public assistance[56] and extends eligibility to comparable groups of *medically indigent persons,* i.e., needy families with dependent children, and blind, disabled or elderly persons who are not on welfare. All *needy children* (under 21) are also made eligible.

The federal share of the program's costs is 53-80 percent, according to a state's per capita income.

Participation in the new medical assistance program is optional for the states, who can elect to continue (until January 1970) under the old medical provisions of the public assistance titles; after January 1970 federal payments for medical care of the medically indigent aged (Kerr-Mills program) will be made only under the new program, which would now have to include the other groups as well. A state not starting the new program by January 1970 may no longer receive federal funds for medical care under the public assistance programs.

In states electing to implement the new program, all persons on public assistance (federally aided categories) are to be included. The same program of services is to be made available to all persons included in the program,

---

[56]Persons eligible for Aid to Families with Dependent Children, Old Age Assistance, Aid to the Blind, and Aid to the Permanently and Totally Disabled.

except that states electing to include aged persons in mental and tuberculosis hospitals are not required to extend the same services to persons under 65.

As a minimum, a medical assistance program must include (at least some of each of) the following:

1. Inpatient hospital services
2. Outpatient hospital services
3. Other laboratory and X-ray services
4. Skilled nursing home services
5. Physicians' services

Additional services which the states could made available are:

6. Medical care furnished by licensed practitioners
7. Home health care services
8. Private duty nursing services
9. Clinic services
10. Dental services
11. Physical therapy and related services
12. Prescribed drugs, dentures, prosthetic devices, and eyeglasses
13. Other diagnostic, screening, preventive, and rehabilitation services
14. Inpatient hospital and skilled nursing home services for individuals 65 or over in tuberculosis or mental hospitals
15. Any other medical care recognized under state law

The states are required to show progress toward broadening the scope of services available and liberalizing the (state's) eligibility requirements for medical assistance with a view toward furnishing, by July 1, 1975, *comprehensive services to substantially all individuals meeting the state's eligibility standards* with regard to income and resources.

No durational residence requirements may be imposed nor any lien against a recipient's property during his lifetime, or lifetime of spouse and surviving minor children. Financial responsibility of relatives other than for spouse or minor children may not be taken into account for purposes of determining eligibility.

Payment for inpatient hospital services is to be made on the basis of *reasonable cost.*

A single state agency is to be designated to administer the medical assistance program except that the determination of eligibility shall be made by the agency administering the program for *old age assistance* (in effect, the state's department of public welfare).

Maternal and Child Health and Crippled Children's Services

There were a number of amendments to Title V:

1. Increased grant funds are authorized for maternal and child health and crippled children's services.
2. Grants are authorized for *training professional personnel* for care of crippled children, particularly children with multiple handicaps.
3. Special Project Grants for Health of School and Preschool Children.[57]

    Grants are authorized for "projects of a comprehensive nature for health care and services for *children and youth* of school age or for preschool children" particularly in areas with concentrations of low income families.

    Grants may be made to a state or local health agency, the agency administering the Title V programs, to any school of medicine (with appropriate participation by a school of dentistry) or to any affiliated teaching hospital.

    Projects are to include at least such screening, diagnosis, preventive services, treatment, correction of defects, and aftercare, both medical and dental, as may be provided for in regulations of the Secretary.

    Treatment, correction of defects, or aftercare provided under the project is to be available only to children *who would not otherwise receive it because they are from low income families* or for other reasons beyond their control.
4. Payments for inpatient hospital services are to be made on the basis of *reasonable costs.*
5. Increased grant funds are authorized for child welfare services.

8. MEDICARE AND MEDICAID AMENDMENTS OF 1966-1971

During 1966 and 1967 there were several short amendments to the Medicare section of the Social Security Act, providing for extension of the initial and first general enrollment periods, and adjusting the reimbursement formula for proprietary extended care facilities.

Social Security Amendments of 1967

    These amendments included a number of changes and adjustments in the Medicare and Medicaid programs:

Medicare Amendments

1. Provision for direct payment to the patient for physicians' services on the basis of an *itemized bill*—not necessarily a receipted (paid) bill.
2. Elimination of the requirement that a physician *certify* to the medical

---

[57]These children and youth projects, and the maternal and infant care projects (1963 Social Security Amendments) have formed the core services of many neighborhood health centers.

necessity of admissions to general hospitals and of outpatient hospital services; (the requirement for periodic certification after admission remains).

3. Inclusion under Part B of the services of *podiatrists* for non-routine foot care.
4. Transfer of hospital *outpatient diagnostic services* from Part A to Part B.
5. Provision for the payment of *full reasonable charges for radiologists' and pathologists' services* to inpatients; (deductible and coinsurance no longer applicable to these services).
6. Provision for purchase of durable medical equipment for use in the home.
7. Inclusion of outpatient *physical therapy* under Part B.
8. Provision for payment under Part B for *diagnostic X-rays* taken in a patient's home or nursing home.
9. Addition of a *lifetime reserve of 60 days* of coverage for inpatient hospital care; (coinsurance of one-half the inpatient deductible).
10. Transfer of the responsibilities of the National Medical Review Committee (members not yet appointed) to the Health Insurance Benefits Advisory Council, which is enlarged to 19 members.

Medicaid Amendments

1. Provision for *limitation of federal participation* in medical assistance payments to families whose income does not exceed 133 percent of the income limit for AFDC payments in any state.
2. For the medically indigent, the states may select the "basic five" services or seven out of the first 14 of the services listed under the original legislation. The states must continue to provide the "basic five" services for public assistance recipients.
3. Requirement, as of July 1969, that the states provide health screening services for Medicaid eligible children and such corrective measures as provided in regulations.
4. If nursing home or hospital services are selected, physicians' services in these institutions are also to be included.
5. Establishment of an *Advisory Council on Medical Assistance,* consisting of 21 persons, to advise the Secretary in matters of administration of the program.
6. Provision that persons covered under medical assistance will have free choice of qualified medical facilities and practitioners.
7. Requirements that skilled nursing homes providing services under the medical assistance program meet the requirements for state licensure, and meet standards similar to those applicable to extended care facilities; that their administration be licensed; and that there be a program of regular medical review of care furnished.

A provision was also included (Title XI) for federal participation in payment for services in *intermediate care* facilities[58] for public assistance recipients.

In 1969, a rider was added to an unrelated bill (PL 91-55) providing for additional modifications of the Medicaid program:

1. Extension to July 1, 1977 of the deadline for states to establish comprehensive medical assistance programs.
2. The states are permitted to reduce some medical services previously available under their medical assistance programs (but prohibiting reduction of cash payments to public assistance recipients).

An additional amendment in 1971 (PL 92-223) broadened the intermediate care facilities provisions to include, optionally, Medicaid recipients other than those on public assistance.

9. SOCIAL SECURITY AMENDMENTS "HR-1" OF 1972*

"An Act to amend the Social Security Act, and for other purposes."

The Social Security Amendments of 1972 made important changes in the Social Security Act, including extensive amendments of the Medicare and Medicaid provisions.

Title 1. Provisions Relating to Old Age, Survivors and Disability Insurance

This title makes a number of adjustments in OASDI provisions for various categories of beneficiaries.

Title II. Provisions Relating to Medicare, Medicaid and Maternal and Child Health

This title incorporates a large number of amendments (97 separate sections) affecting Medicare and Medicaid, many addressed to the control of costs, many making significant changes. Notable among the provisions are the following:[59]

---

[58] An institution providing a level of care beyond room and board, but not of a degree required of a skilled nursing home.

*PL 92-603.

[59] Briefly summarized.

Health Insurance for the Disabled. Persons who have received cash benefits under the disability insurance provisions of the Social Security Act for at least 24 months will be eligible for medical benefits under Title XVIII of the Social Security Act (which will now read *Health Insurance for the Aged and Disabled*).

Part B Premiums, Deductibles and Automatic Enrollment. Part B premiums will not be increased more than the most recent percentage increase in social security cash benefits. Beneficiaries will be automatically enrolled upon entitlement with provision made for those who wish to decline enrollment. The annual deductible is increased to $60.

Cost Sharing Under Medicaid. (1) The states must charge an income-related enrollment fee to medically indigent persons included under Medicaid programs, and may charge nominal deductibles and co-payments; (2) The states may charge public assistance recipients nominal deductibles and co-payments for other than the basic mandated services.

Deferred Loss of Medicaid Due to Increased Earnings. Families who lose Medicaid eligibility because of increased earnings will remain covered for four months.

Limitation of Payments for Unnecessary Capital Expenditures. Payment will not be made for capital expenditures which have been disapproved by State or local planning agencies.

Experiments and Demonstrations Related to Increased Economy and Efficiency of Health Services. Grants and contracts are authorized for studies, experiments and demonstrations related to prospective reimbursement; the three-day hospitalization requirement for skilled nursing home admission; ambulatory surgical centers, intermediate care facilities; home health and day care services; payment for services of physician's assistants and nurse practitioners; and use of clinical psychologists.

Health Maintenance Organizations. Single annual per capita payments may be made to health maintenance organizations[60] for Part A and Part B services provided to or arranged for Medicare beneficiaries. Such organizations must provide care to a group of enrollees of whom at least one half are not

---

[60]The definition of such organizations includes (1) provision, either directly or through arrangements, of services to enrolled individuals on the basis of a predetermined periodic rate regardless of the frequency or extent of services and (2) provision of services primarily through such organization's physicians or under arrangements with groups of physicians (in group or individual practice) which are reimbursed on the basis of an aggregate fixed sum or per capita basis.

Medicare beneficiaries. Up to 20 percent of any savings made by a health maintenance organization relative to the per capita annual costs of services to non-HMO enrollees will be divided equally between the organization and the Medicare trust funds.

Payment of Teaching Physicians.   Payment under Part B for services of physicians in hospital teaching programs will generally be made on a cost basis only except for bona fide private patients. Payment for donated services of such physicians will be made to a fund designated for charitable or educational purposes.

Advance Approval of Skilled Nursing Facility and Home Health Benefits.   Minimum periods of presumed eligibility for post-hospital services may be established by the Secretary.

Elimination of Requirement of Progressively More Comprehensive Medicaid Programs.   The Title IX section requiring that the states progress toward the provision of comprehensive Medicaid services by July 1, 1977 is repealed.

Level of State Medicaid Funding.   The Title IX section prohibiting a state from reducing its aggregate payments for Medicaid services is repealed.

Payments to States for Claims and Information Systems.   Matching funds may be paid to the states for development and installation of claims processing and information retrieval systems (90 percent of costs) and, under certain conditions, for their operation (75 percent of costs).

Utilization Review Under Medicaid and Child Health Programs. Hospitals and skilled nursing facilities participating in Medicaid or child health programs must, with some exceptions, use the same utilization review committees as are used under the Medicare program.

Validation of Joint Commission on Accreditation of Hospitals Surveys. Arrangements are authorized for the state Medicare certifying agencies to survey, by sampling, participating hospitals which have been accredited by the Joint Commission on Hospital Accreditation. The Secretary may in addition prescribe higher standards than required for accreditation by the Commission.

Conformation of Skilled Care Services and Facilities Under Medicare and Medicaid.   Skilled care services are similarly defined with respect to both

Medicare and Medicaid, and standards of skilled nursing facilities are to be the same under both programs. The term *extended care facility* is eliminated. [61]

Professional Standards Review. This is the most extensive and important of the provisions directed to the problems of cost and quality control and medical necessity of services.[62] A new part (B) *Professional Standards Review* is added to Title XI of the Social Security Act. Provision is made for the establishment of *Professional Standards Review Organizations* within states for the review of the professional activities of physicians and other practitioners, and institutional and other providers of services in designated geographical areas.[63] These organizations are to be associations of physicians and open to and representative of physicians in the area. (After January 1, 1976, and then only if there is no such organization meeting the specified conditions, other competent agencies or organizations may be designated.)

Statewide Professional Standards Review Councils and a National Professional Standards Review Council are also to be established.

Social Services in Skilled Nursing Facilities. It is no longer to be required under Medicare that medical social services be furnished in a skilled nursing facility.

Chiropractic Services. Chiropractors' services are covered under Medicare and Medicaid with respect to treatment by means of manual manipulation of the spine; in the case of Medicare, this is specifically to be for correction of a subluxation demonstrated by X-ray.

Speech Pathology Services. Speech pathology is covered as a part of outpatient physical therapy services under Medicare.

Termination of Medical Assistance Advisory Council. The Medical Assistance Advisory Council is terminated and its Title IX advisory functions added to those of the Health Insurance Benefits Advisory Council.

Review of Care in Intermediate Care Facilities. The requirements for professional review of care and placement of patients are extended to intermediate care facilities.

---

[61] Extended care facilities are now termed *skilled nursing facilities.*

[62] The declared purpose of this section is to assure "that the services for which payment may be made under the Social Security Act will conform to appropriate professional standards and that payment for such services will be made—(1) only when, and to the extent, medically necessary . . ." and (2) in the case of inpatient services, only when these cannot "effectively be provided on an outpatient basis or more economically in a health care facility of a different type."

[63] The review of services provided other than in institutions will be at the option of the organization and subject to the approval of the Secretary.

Psychiatric Hospital Care for Individuals Under 21. Inpatient psychiatric hospital services under Medicaid are extended, under specified conditions, to persons under age 21.

Public Information concerning Survey Reports. The pertinent findings of surveys of health care institutions and agencies with regard to compliance with conditions of participation under Medicare are to be made available to the public.

Family Planning Services. Family planning services are added to the basic services which must be made available under Medicaid.

Penalty for Failure to Provide Child Health Screening under Medicaid. The matching funds to the states under Medicaid will be reduced by 1 percent where the states do not implement the previous requirements for providing for child health screening and subsequent corrective treatment services for children in families receiving aid to dependent children.[64]

Home Health Services Coinsurance. Coinsurance payments for home health services under Part B are eliminated.

Treatment for Chronic Renal Disease. Persons insured under Social Security, and their dependents, who require hemodialysis or renal transplantation for chronic renal disease are deemed disabled for purpose of coverage under Title XVIII, beginning 3 months after initiation of a course of renal dialysis. Reimbursement is to be limited to treatment centers meeting specified requirements.

Title III. Supplemental Security Income
For the Aged, Blind and Disabled
This title creates, effective January 1, 1974, a new federal minimum income program (under a new Title XVI) to replace the federally aided adult public assistance programs. Grants to the states for social services for these groups will be continued under a new Title VI. (No change is made in the federal-state programs of aid to families with dependent children.)

Title IV. Miscellaneous
This title includes provision for increased grants to the states for child welfare services.

---

[64] The programs established under these provisions have come to be known as Early and Periodic Screening, Diagnosis and Treatment (EPSDT) programs.

10. SUMMARY OF MEDICARE

Title XVIII. Health Insurance for the Aged *and disabled.*

Part A—Hospital Insurance

Benefits
Hospital Inpatient Services
Up to 90 days during any spell of illness.[65] Deductible ($84) and coinsurance ($21 per day after the sixtieth hospital day).[66]
60-day lifetime reserve ($42 coinsurance)[66]
90-day lifetime limit for inpatient psychiatric care
Post-Hospital Extended Care Services[67]
Up to 100 days during any spell of illness. Coinsurance ($10.50 per day[66] after the twentieth day.)
Three-day prior hospital admission required
Continuing *skilled nursing care* or other skilled rehabilitation services must be needed for a condition for which the preceding inpatient services were received.
Post-Hospital Home Health Services
Up to 100 visits in a one-year period, and related services and supplies
Skilled nursing care or physical or speech therapy must be needed for a condition for which the inpatient services were received. Services to be rendered under a plan established and periodically reviewed by a physician.
Beneficiary must be essentially confined to the home

Exclusions—Private Duty Nurses

Financing—Cost of First Three Pints of Blood
A special earnings tax on employees, employers and self-employed persons
Conditions of Participation
Include *utilization review plans* for hospitals and skilled nursing facilities

---

[65] Also referred to as a "benefit period."
[66] Deductible and coinsurance figures as of January 1, 1974.
[67] In a skilled nursing facility.

Part B—Supplementary Medical Insurance

Benefits

Physicians' Services

Services of doctors of medicine and osteopathy, including professional services of hospital-based specialists (radiologists and pathologists)

Limited, specified services by dentists, podiatrists, optometrists and chiropractors

Hospital Outpatient Services

Diagnostic Procedures
Laboratory and X-ray services
Home Health Services

Up to 100 visits in a one-year period. Conditions essentially the same as for Part A services, except for prior hospitalization.

Outpatient Physical Therapy and Speech Pathology Services

Services rendered under the direct supervision of a physician or under certain circumstances as a part of home health services.

Other Medical and Health Services

Supplies, equipment, prostheses, radiation therapy, ambulance services (only, and under limited conditions, to a hospital or skilled nursing facility)

Deductibles and Coinsurance

Deductible is $60 per year; coinsurance is 20 percent of charges. (No deductible or coinsurance for home health services or radiologists' and pathologists' services to inpatients.)

Exclusions

Glasses, dentures, hearing aids, drugs, check-ups, dental care, routine foot care

$250 annual limit on out of hospital psychiatric services

Financing

Monthly premium ($6.30) plus government matching

II. SUMMARY OF MEDICAID

Title XIX. Grants to States for Medical Assistance Programs

Federal matching grants are made available, at the option of the states, for a single medical assistance program for:

1. Recipients of federally aided public assistance[68]
2. Recipients of supplemental security income benefits
3. Medically indigent in comparable groups (families with dependent children, as defined for purposes of public assistance, and the aged, blind and disabled)
4. Other needy children

States participating in the Medicaid program must include both categories 1 and 2 above.

Programs are to include (some of each of) five basic services[69]

1. Inhospital services
2. Outpatient hospital services
3. Other laboratory and X-ray services
4. Skilled nursing home services
5. Physicians' services

Also to be included by each participating state are:

1. A program for screening of children for defects and chronic conditions, and appropriate treatment
2. Family planning services

Federal matching: 50-83 percent of costs (according to state's per capita income)

All states except Arizona have established Medicaid programs.

Administration. Social and Rehabilitation Service (Medical Assistance Administration)

---

[68]Prior to January 1, 1974, the federally aided public assistance groups were families with dependent children (children deprived of parental support due to death, absence or incapacity of a parent, or, in certain circumstances, unemployment of the father), and indigent aged, blind, and disabled. The latter three groups are now under the federal supplemental security income program.

[69]Alternatively, (for medically indigent) states could select seven among these and other services (See p. 135). States including skilled nursing home services must also include home health services.

State Agency—usually the department of public welfare

Advisory Council—Health Insurance Benefits Advisory Council

12.   SUMMARY OF THE SOCIAL SECURITY ACT TITLES

Title   I.   Grants to States for Old Age Assistance and Medical Assistance for the Aged (Repealed)*

Title   II.   Federal Old Age, Survivors and Disability Insurance Benefits (OASDI)

Benefits (monthly cash payments) were extended to dependents and survivors in 1939, and to disabled workers (at age 50) in 1956; the age limit for disability was removed in 1960.

Title   III.   Grants to States for Unemployment Compensation Administration

Title   IV.   Grants to States for Aid and Services to Needy Families with Children and for Child Welfare Services

Child welfare provisions were placed under this Title in 1967 (from Title V).

Title   V.   Maternal and Child Health and Crippled Children's Services

Title   VI.   Grants to States for Services to the Aged, Blind, or Disabled*

Title   VII.   Administration

Provides for the administration of the Act by the Secretary of HEW and the Commissioner of Social Security. (The Social Security Board was abolished in 1946 and its functions transferred to the newly established Social Security Administration in the Federal Security Agency.) This Title also authorizes training grants for public welfare personnel.

Title   VIII.   Taxes with Respect to Employment

(These provisions are now in the Internal Revenue Code)

Title   IX.   Miscellaneous Provisions Relating to   Employment Security

Title   X.   Grants to States for Aid to the Blind (Repealed)*

Title   XI.   General Provisions and Professional Standards Review (1972)

Title   XII.   Advances to States, Unemployment Funds (1944)

Title   XIII.   Reconversion Unemployment Benefits for Seamen   (1946) (Expired)

Title   XIV.   Grants to States for Aid to the Permanently and Totally Disabled (1950) (Repealed)*

Title   XV.   Unemployment Compensation for Federal Employees and the Ex-Servicemen's Unemployment Compensation Program (1954), 1958) (Repealed)

These provisions are codified elsewhere.

Title   XVI.   Supplemental Security Income for the Aged, Blind, and Disabled (1972)*

Title XVII.   Grants for Planning Comprehensive Action to Combat Mental Retardation (1963) (Expired)

Title XVIII. Health Insurance for the Aged and Disabled (1965, 1972) "Medicare"

Title XIX.   Grants to States for Medical Assistance Programs (1965) "Medicaid"

*Prior to January 1, 1974, there were four federally aided public assistance ("welfare") categories under titles I, IV, X and XIV: Old Age Assistance (OAA), Aid to Families with Dependent Children (AFDC), Aid to the Blind (AB) and Aid to the Permanently and Totally Disabled (APTD).

Under provisions of the 1972 Social Security Amendments (see p. 142) the three adult assistance categories (OAA, AB, APTD) became part of a new federal income supplement program (*Supplemental Security Income,* SSI) under a new Title VI. Titles I, X and XIV were repealed. Grants to the states for social services for the aged, blind and disabled were continued under a new Title VI. (The original provisions of Title VI, Public Health Work, had been transferred to the Public Health Service Act in 1944.)

Administration of the Social Security Act (federal level)

OASDI program—*Social Security Administration*

Public Assistance and Medical Assistance (Medicaid) - *Social and Rehabilitation Service*

Medicare - *Social Security Administration* and *Office of Professional Standards Review*

Maternal and Child Health - *Health Services Administration*

Unemployment Insurance - *Department of Labor*

Supplemental Security Income - *Social Security Administration*

References

Social Security Programs in the United States. U.S. Department of Health, Education, and Welfare-Social Security Administration. This is an excellent summary of programs related to the Social Security Act. It is revised periodically, following major amendments.

Basic Readings in Social Security U.S. Department of Health, Education and Welfare, Social Security Administration, Office of Research and Statistics, 1973, a good bibliography on the subject of Social Security.

13. THE PUBLIC HEALTH SERVICE ACT

An Act to consolidate and revise the laws relating to the Public Health Service and for other purposes.

The Public Health Service Act of 1944 revised and brought together in one statute all existing legislation concerning the Public Health Service (including

Title VI of the Social Security Act). It set forth provisions for the organization, staffing, and activities of the Service. It has subsequently been the vehicle, by amendment, of a number of important federal grant-in-aid programs.

Title I. Short Title and Definitions
Titles I through V may be cited as the "Public Health Service Act."

Title II. Administration
General organization of the Public Health Service. It shall be administered by the Surgeon General under the direction of the Federal Security Administrator. The Service shall consist of: (1) the Office of the Surgeon General, (2) the National Institute of Health, (3) the Bureau of Medical Services, and (4) the Bureau of State Services.

Grades, ranks, and titles of the Commissioned Corps, and relevant policies and regulations.[70]

Organization and duties of the National Advisory Health Council and National Advisory Cancer Council.

Title III. General Powers and Duties of the Public Health Service

Part A. Research and Investigations

Sec. 301   The Service shall conduct, encourage, cooperate in, and promote research and investigations relating to physical and mental diseases and impairments.

Sec. 302   In carrying out the purposes of this section with regard to narcotics, activities shall include studies and investigations regarding the use and misuse of narcotic drugs. The Surgeon General shall give aid and advice to state officials in the care, treatment, and rehabilitation of narcotics addicts.

Part B. Federal-State Cooperation

Sec. 311   The Surgeon General is authorized to accept from and provide *assistance to state and local authorities* in prevention and control of communicable diseases.

Sec. 312   A *health conference* of the state health authorities shall be called annually.[71]

---

[70]Commissioned officers include personnel in "medicine, surgery, dentistry, hygiene, sanitary engineering, pharmacy, nursing, or related scientific specialties in public health."

[71]Known as the Conference of State and Territorial Health Officers.

Sec. 313 Collection and compilation of *vital statistics.*

Sec. 314 Grants and services to the states to assist in *venereal disease control, tuberculosis control,* and the establishment and maintenance of adequate *state and local public health services.*

   Annual allotments to the states shall be made on the basis of: (1) population, (2) the size of the venereal disease and tuberculosis problems and other special health problems and (3) the financial need of the respective states.

   Grants shall be paid on the condition that the states spend for the same general purpose from its funds an amount determined in accordance with regulations.

   Regulations and amendments regarding grants to the states shall be made after consultation with a conference of the state health authorities; the Surgeon General shall obtain insofar as practicable the agreement of the state health authorities prior to the issuance of such regulations or amendments.

Sec. 315 The Surgeon General shall issue from time to time *information related to public health,* including publications for the public, weekly reports on health conditions, and other pertinent information for those engaged in work related to the functions of the Service.

Part C. Hospitals, Medical Examinations, and Medical Care

Sec. 322 Management and operation of the institutions, hospitals, and stations of the Service. Medical care to be provided for *merchant seamen* and certain other persons.[72]

Sec. 323 The Service is to furnish medical services in *penal and correctional* institutions of the United States.

Sec. 324 The Surgeon General is authorized to provide medical services to *federal employees* and longshoremen for work-related illness or injury and medical examinations for employees and retirees.

Sec. 325 Medical examination of *aliens.*

Sec. 326 Members of the Coast Guard, Coast and Geodetic Survey and the Commissioned Corps of the Public Health Service are entitled to *treatment and hospitalization by the Service.*

Part D. Lepers

Sec. 331- The Public Health Service shall receive and care for persons with
332 leprosy.

---

[72]Including members of the U.S. Maritime Service, Merchant Marine cadets, quarantine and immigration detainees.

Part E. Narcotics Addicts

Sec. 341-   Care and treatment, in hospitals of the Service, of narcotics addicts
345   who are federal prisoners or who voluntarily request treatment.

Part F. Biological Products

Sec. 351-   Regulation of the manufacture, labeling, and sale of biological
352   products (virus, serum, toxin, anti-toxin, or other product) applicable to the prevention or cure of disease or injuries of man.

Part G. Quarantine and Inspection

Sec. 361-   Inspection, quarantine, and other procedures necessary to prevent
367   transmission or spread of communicable diseases from foreign countries into states or possessions or from one state or possession into
another.

Title IV. National Cancer Institute[73]

The National Cancer Institute shall be a division of the National
Institute of Health, to carry out the purposes of Part A of Title III (Research
and Investigation) with regard to cancer. It is to:

1. Conduct and assist researches, investigations and studies relating to the cause,
   prevention and treatment of cancer.
2. Promote the coordination of researches conducted by the Institute and
   similar researches conducted by other agencies and individuals.
3. Provide training and instruction in technical matters relating to diagnoses
   and treatment of cancer.
4. Provide fellowships in the Institute.
5. Secure for the Institute consultation service and advice of cancer experts
   from the United States and abroad.
6. Cooperate with state health agencies in prevention, control and eradication
   of cancer.
7. Procure, use, and lend radium for purposes of this Title.

Grants-in-aid for cancer projects shall be made only after review and
recommendations of the National Cancer Advisory Council.

This Title is not to be construed as limiting the functions or authority
of the Surgeon General or the Public Health Service under any other Title of this
Act relating to the study of the prevention, diagnosis and treatment of cancer.

---

[73] This title in effect re-enacted the National Cancer Act of 1937.

Title V. Miscellaneous

Miscellaneous regulations, and authorization for the *admission to St. Elizabeths Hospital* of insane patients entitled to treatment by the Service.

Title VI. Temporary and Emergency Provisions and Amendments and Repeals

Amendments

There have been many amendments to the Public Health Service Act. Several are of particular interest:

The *Hospital Survey and Construction Act of 1946* (Hill-Burton Act) inaugurated the Hill-Burton program of health facilities construction.

The *Health Amendments of 1956* (grants for training in public health and nursing) initiated the program of federal assistance for education and training of health personnel which has been gradually extended and broadened by subsequent legislation to many categories of health personnel and institutions.

The *Heart Disease, Cancer and Stroke Amendments of 1965* established the Regional Medical Programs.

The *Comprehensive Health Planning Amendments of 1966* ("Partnership for Health") were designed to give the states more flexibility in use of their grants-in-aid for public health work, and to encourage comprehensive health planning; it is the base for the state and areawide comprehensive health planning "A" and "B" agencies.

The *Health Maintenance Organization Act of 1973* established a program of financial assistance for the development of health maintenance organizations.

These amendments are described more fully in the following sections. Other noteworthy amending Acts are:

Health Services for Agricultural Migratory Workers (1962). This Act established a program of grants for family clinics and other health services for migrant workers.

Communicable Disease Control Amendments of 1970. This legislation re-established the categorical grant program for control of communicable diseases, including tuberculosis, venereal disease, rubella, measles, Rh disease, poliomyelitis, diphtheria, tetanus and whooping cough.

Family Planning Services and Population Research Act of 1970. This established an Office of Population Affairs under the Assistant Secretary for Health and Scientific Affairs. It added Title X, *Population Research and Voluntary Family Planning Programs,* to the Public Health Service Act. This authorized project, formula and training grants and contracts for family planning programs and services (abortion excepted), and research grants and contracts in fields related to family planning and population.

Emergency Health Personnel Act of 1970. This Act authorized the Secretary to assign commissioned officers and other health personnel of the Public Health Service to areas designated as in critical need of health manpower. It provided a statutory base for the National Health Service Corps.

National Sickle Cell Anemia Control Act (1972). This added a new Title XI to the Public Health Service Act: *Sickle Cell Anemia Program.* It authorized grants and contracts for screening and counseling, research, and informational programs related to sickle cell anemia.

National Cooley's Anemia Control Act (1972). Title XI was changed to *Genetic Blood Disorders* and Part B, *Cooley's Anemia Programs,* was added. This authorized grants and contracts for Cooley's anemia screening, treatment and counseling, research, and educational programs.

Communicable Disease Control Amendments of 1972. This Act extended the programs of grants for communicable disease control and established a separate one for prevention and control of venereal disease.

Health Programs Extension Act of 1973. This Act extended through June 30, 1974 a number of programs whose authorizations were due to expire. These included migrant health, comprehensive health planning, Hill-Burton, allied health manpower training, regional medical programs and family planning programs as well as programs under the Community Mental Health Centers Act and the Developmental Disabilities Services and Facilities Construction Act.

Emergency Medical Services Systems Act of 1973. This added a new title to the Public Health Service Act: Title XII—*Emergency Medical Services Systems.* It established a program of grants and contracts for the development and improvement of area emergency medical services systems, and for related research and training.

14. HOSPITAL SURVEY AND CONSTRUCTION ACT OF 1946* "HILL-BURTON ACT"

> An Act to amend the Public Health Service Act to authorize grants to the States for surveying their hospital and public health centers and for planning construction of additional facilities, and to authorize grants to assist in such construction.

*PL 79-725

This Act established the first of the many post-World War II federally aided health programs.

Background

There was relatively little hospital construction during the years of the Great Depression and World War II. In 1944 a Commission on Hospital Care was organized by the American Hospital Association and the Public Health Service to study the national need for hospital facilities. The principles developed by the Commission and the Public Health Service are reflected in the Survey and Construction Act, introduced by Senators Hill and Burton, which became Title VI of the Public Health Service Act.

Summary of Major Provisions[74]

1. Grants to assist the states to *inventory* their existing hospitals and health centers and to *survey* the need and develop programs for the construction of such facilities.
2. Grants to the states for *construction projects.*
3. Federal funds for surveys and planning to be allotted to the states on the *basis of population.* Within its allotment, a state may receive a grant equal to 33-1/3 percent of these expenses.

    Funds for construction to be allotted annually to the states in accordance with a *formula* based on population and per capita income; from this allotment, grants may be made covering 33-1/3 percent of the cost of construction projects.
4. In order to receive funds, a state must (among other provisions):
    a. Designate a *single state agency* to administer or supervise administration of the program, and establish a *state advisory council* to consult with the state agency. The council to include representatives of nongovernmental agencies and state agencies concerned with hospitals, and representatives of the *consumers* of hospital services.
    b. Submit a *state plan* for the construction of facilities based on the state-wide survey of need and conforming to regulations prescribed by the Surgeon General.
5. The Surgeon General shall develop regulations prescribing:
    a. The number of general hospital beds required to provide adequate hospital services in a state and the general methods by which such beds would be distributed. (Total beds for any state not to exceed 4.5 per thousand population, except up to 5.5 beds per thousand in less populated states.)

---

[74] The general language of this Act is representative of legislation authorizing grants-in-aid to the states.

    b. The number of tuberculosis, mental disease, and chronic disease hospital beds required, and their distribution.

    c. The number and distribution of public health centers.

    d. The general manner in which the state agency will determine priorities for projects within a state, with special consideration to be given to hospital serving *rural communities.*

    e. General *standards* for construction and equipment for hospitals.

6. Grants are to be available only to states who enact or have enacted legislation providing for minimum standards of maintenance and operation for hospitals receiving federal aid under this program.

7. The Surgeon General is to consult with a *Federal Hospital Council* in administration of this title. The council shall consist of eight members (plus the Surgeon General), including four representatives of consumers of hospital services.

By 1949, all the states and territories had had state plans approved by the Surgeon General. In most instances, the state health department had been designated as the responsible agency for the administration of the program. Most states now had licensure laws, most of which were applicable to all hospitals, not just those eligible for federal aid.

Hill-Burton Amendments

The Hill-Burton Act has been amended frequently since its original enactment.

The *Hospital Survey and Construction Amendments of 1949* extended the program, increased the authorized funds and provided that the federal share of the costs of construction projects could be as much as 66-2/3 percent, depending on the relative need and economic status of the area involved. Additionally, grants were authorized for *research and demonstrations* relating to the development, utilization and coordination of hospital services and facilities.[75]

The *Medical Facilities Survey and Construction Act of 1954* authorized grants for surveys and for construction of *diagnostic and treatment* centers (including hospital OPDs), *chronic disease* hospitals, rehabilitation facilities and nursing homes.

Chronic disease hospitals were already included in the existing program, as were the other types of facilities when part of a hospital. The purpose of this legislation was to encourage the construction of such facilities by specifically earmarking funds for them and by including them though not part of a hospital.

The *Community Health Services and Facilities Act of 1961,* which dealt primarily with the question of improving out of hospital services

---

[75]However, no funds were actually appropriated under this authorization until 1956.

for the aged and chronically ill, included several amendments to the Hill-Burton program. Funds for *nursing home* construction were increased and the hospital research and demonstration grant program was extended to other medical facilities.

The *Hospital and Medical Facilities Amendments of 1964* extended the program and authorized grants specifically earmarked for *modernization* of hospitals with more priority being given to urban areas.[76]

A new category of long-term care facilities was created which combined the chronic disease hospitals and nursing home categories, and its funding authorization was increased.

A state was now permitted to use up to 2 percent of its allotment (up to $50,000) for half the *costs of administration* of the program.

Grants were authorized to the state agencies for up to 50 percent of the costs of comprehensive regional or local area *plans* for coordination of existing and planned health facilities. (Planning to be done by state agencies or by designated local public or nonprofit groups.

Language was added requiring that "any facility or portion thereof to be constructed or modernized, [is] to be made available to all persons residing in the territorial area of the applicant." This replaced the previous "separate . . . if like quality" provisions.[77]

The *Medical Facilities Construction and Modernization Amendments of 1970*[78] again extended the program and added new provisions for federal loans and loan guarantees for construction and modernization. A new program of project grants was established for emergency rooms, communications networks, and transportation systems.

Administration
Health Resources Administration (Health Care Facilities Service)

15. HEART DISEASE, CANCER AND STROKE AMENDMENTS OF 1965;*" REGIONAL MEDICAL PROGRAMS"

An Act to amend the Public Health Service Act to assist in combatting heart disease, cancer, stroke, and related diseases.

This legislation reflects the general goals expressed in the 1964 report of the President's Commission on Heart Disease, Cancer and Stroke, although the recommendations were much modified.

---

*PL 89-239

[76] Authority for modernization existed in previous legislation but priority was given to "hospitals serving rural communities and areas with relatively small financial resources."

[77] A federal court had ruled (1963) this clause unconstitutional (Moses H. Cone Memorial Hospital *vs.* Simkins); the Supreme Court refused (1964) to review this decision, thus in effect barring racial segregation in hospitals receiving federal funds under the Hill-Burton program.

[78] Passed over Presidential veto.

The purposes of this title are:

1. ". . . to encourage and assist in the establishment of regional cooperative arrangements among medical schools, research institutions, and hospitals for research and training (including continuing education) and for related demonstrations of patient care in the fields of heart disease, cancer, stroke and related diseases;
2. "to afford the medical profession and the medical institutions of the nation, through such cooperative arrangements, the opportunity of making available to their patients the latest advances in the diagnosis and treatment of these diseases,
3. ". . . and to accomplish these ends without interfering with the patterns, or the methods of financing, of patient care or professional practice or with the administration of hospitals. . ."

Summary of Major Provisions

Grants are authorized to assist universities, medical schools, research institutions and other institutions and agencies in *planning* the development of regional medical programs and in *establishment and operation* of such programs.

A *regional medical program* is defined as a cooperative arrangement among a group of institutions or agencies engaged in research, training, diagnosis and treatment relating to heart disease, cancer or stroke, and, at the option of the applicant, related diseases. This group must:

1. Be situated within an appropriate geographic area (which may be composed of part or parts of one or more states)
2. Consist of one or more medical centers, one or more clinical research centers, and one or more hospitals [79]
3. Have in effect adequate cooperative arrangements

An applicant must designate an *advisory group* to advise the applicant (and the participating institutions and agencies) regarding the planning and operation of the regional medical program. The advisory group is to include practicing physicians, medical center officials, hospital administrators, and representatives from appropriate organizations and institutions.

---

[79] "A *medical center* means a medical school or other medical institution involved in postgraduate medical training and one or more affiliated hospitals."

A *clinical research center* means an institution (or part of an institution) the primary function of which is research and training of specialists and which, in connection therewith, provides specialized diagnostic and treatment services.

A *hospital* means "a health facility in which local capability for diagnosis and treatment is supported and augmented by the program established under this title."

A *National Advisory Council on Regional Medical Programs* is established to consist of the Surgeon General and 12 other members. At least two are to be practicing physicians, one outstanding in the study, diagnosis and treatment of cancer and one outstanding in the study, diagnosis, and treatment of stroke.

Regional Medical Programs Amendments

The *Public Health Service Amendments* of *1968* extended the regional medical programs and made a number of adjustments and clarifications, such as:

1. Extension of the program to Guam, American Samoa and Trust Territory of the Pacific Islands
2. Membership of the National Advisory Countil increased to 16
3. Specific provision that *federal hospitals* may participate in regional medical programs
4. Authorized the use of up to 1 percent of the annual appropriation for *evaluation* of the program [80]

More extensive additions and changes were made in the *Public Health Service Amendments of 1970.* These extended the program for three years and (among other provisions):

1. Broadened the scope of the program by adding *kidney disease* as one of the diseases to which the program is specifically addressed; Title IX now to read " . . . Stroke, Kidney Disease and Other Related Diseases."
2. Further broadened and clarified the purposes of the Title:
   a. To explicitly include *medical data exchange* among the activities of the programs
   b. To make explicit that *prevention* and *rehabilitation* as well as diagnosis and treatment are program concerns
   c. "To promote and foster linkages among health care institutions and providers so as to strengthen and improve *primary care* and the relationship between specialized and primary care"
   d. "To improve health services for persons residing in areas with limited health services"
3. Required official health and *health planning* agency representation on the *advisory groups* and that public members include persons familiar with the financing of, as well as the need for, services and that such public members be sufficient in numbers to insure adequate community orientation of regional medical programs.

---

[80] The practice of earmarking funds for evaluation was subsequently extended to other grant-in-aid programs.

4. Required that the appropriate regional metropolitan or local *areawide comprehensive health planning agency* (authorized under Section 314b)[81] have an opportunity to consider (for example, review and comment on) any operational grant proposal or application of a regional medical program involving facilities, services or functions within that areawide agency's jurisdiction.

5. Designated the *Assistant Secretary of Health and Scientific Affairs* as chairman of the National Advisory Council on Regional Medical Programs and increased the size of the Council to 20 members.

6. Provided specific *contract*[82] as well as grant authority in carrying out the purposes of the legislation.

7. Authorized *training grants* for training health manpower in the areas included in the legislation, and permitted support of research, studies, investigations and demonstrations designed to maximize the utilization of manpower in the deliver of health services.

8. Specifically permitted funds to be used for special projects for improving and developing new means for the *delivery of health services* concerned with heart disease, cancer, stroke, kidney disease, and other related diseases.

By 1971 there were 56 regional medical programs covering all the states and trust territories. Most encompassed single states but one incorporated two or more states, parts of two or more states, or parts of single states.[83]

Administration
Health Resources Administration (Regional Medical Programs Service)

Note
The regional medical program is among a number of grant-in-aid programs whose continuation is, at the time of this writing, the subject of disagreement between the President and the Congress. It is generally anticipated that this program will not be continued beyond June 30, 1974.

16. COMPREHENSIVE HEALTH PLANNING AND PUBLIC HEALTH SERVICE AMENDMENTS OF 1966;* "PARTNERSHIP FOR HEALTH"

An Act to amend the Public Health Service Act to promote and assist in the extension and improvement of comprehensive health

---

[82]The use of the contract mechanism for federal funding of health related studies, research, and other activities has become common in recent years.

[83]For example, Tri-State Regional Medical Program (Massachusetts, New Hampshire, and Rhode Island), Intermountain Regional Medical Program (Utah and parts of Colorado, Idaho, Montana, Nevada, and Wyoming), and Western New York Regional Medical Program.

*PL 89-749

planning and public health services, [and] to provide for a more effective use of available Federal funds for such planning and services . . .

Background

In the years since the passage of the Public Health Service Act of 1944 the program of grants to the states for public health work had been expended largely by designating funds for specific purposes. As of 1966, most of the federal support to the states for public health services was made available through one or another of such "categorical grants."[84] This system had come under considerable criticism, as being excessively rigid, denying the state health department freedom to determine the allocation ot these funds to public health problems. This legislation represents a departure from this approach to funding of public health services; it authorizes "block" grants for public health programs and includes provisions for the development of state and local planning for comprehensive health services.

These amendments essentially involved a complete revision of Section 314 (Title III) of the Public Health Service Act, which thereafter referred to grants for *Comprehensive Health Planning* and for *Comprehensive Public Health Services.*

Sec. 314a *Grants to the States for Comprehensive State Health Planning*

In order to qualify for these funds, a state is to submit a "plan for comprehensive state health planning." This plan must designate a state agency (new or existing) to be responsible for the state's health planning functions, and provide for the establishment of a *state health planning* council to advise this agency. The council is to include representatives of state and local agencies, nongovernmental organizations and groups, and consumers of health services; a majority of the membership are to be representatives of consumers.

The plan further is to provide for "encouraging cooperative efforts among governmental or nongovernmental agencies, organizations and groups concerned with health services, facilities, or manpower," and for cooperative efforts between them and similar agencies, organizations, and groups in the fields of education, welfare, and rehabilitation.

Sec. 314b *Project Grants for Areawide Health Planning*

Grants are authorized, with the consent of the above state agency, to any other public or nonprofit agency or organization "for developing comprehensive regional, metropolitan area or other local area plans for coordination of existing and planned health services, including facilities and persons required for provision of such services."[85]

Federal share: 75 percent of the costs of such projects.

---

[84] Among these were cancer, chronic illness, dental disease, heart disease, mental illness, tuberculosis, and venereal disease.

[85] The state planning agency is known as the "A" agency; the sub-state agency is known as the "B" or "areawide" agency (or, "314a" and "314b" agencies).

Sec. 314c *Project Grants for Training, Studies, and Demonstrations*

Grants to agencies, institutions, or other organizations for projects for training, studies and demonstrations relating to the development of improved or more effective comprehensive health planning.

Sec. 314d   *Grants for Comprehensive Public Health Services*

Grants to "assist the states in establishing and maintaining adequate public health services, including the training of personnel for state and local health work." Again to qualify for these funds, state plans for the provision of public health services are required and these plans are to be developed in accordance with the plan for comprehensive health planning. The federal share for public health programs under this section is to be 33 1/3 to 66 2/3 percent, and at least 15 percent of a state's allotment is to be used for mental health services.

Sec. 314e   *Project Grants for Health Services Development*[86]

Grants are authorized to public or nonprofit private agencies, institutions or organizations to cover part of the cost of

1. Providing services to meet health needs of limited geographic scope or of specialized regional or national significance;
2. Stimulating and supporting, for an initial period, new programs of health services;
3. Undertaking studies, demonstrations or training designed to develop new methods or improve existing methods of providing health services

Comprehensive Health Planning Amendments

The *Partnership for Health Amendments of 1967* extended the program and made several additions and modifications including:

1. State plans for comprehensive health planning are to provide for assisting each state health institution to develop a program for capital expenditures for replacement, modernization and expansion consistent with meeting the needs of the state for facilities and services most economically, efficiently, and without duplication.
2. Representation of the *interests of local government* in areawide planning agencies is required.
3. After July 1, 1968, 70 percent of the states' grant funds must be available for *services in communities* of the states (i.e., locally).

---

[86]The intent of this section, also, was to provide more flexibility in the use of such project grants than had formerly been the case.

The *Public Health Service Amendments of 1970* extended the program for an additional three years and made several further modifications:

1. State and areawide plans must include *home health services.*
2. The state planning agency could receive a grant under Section 314b if no application for a grant for the region involved has been filed by any other qualified organization.
3. Areawide health planning councils are to be established to include representatives of the interests of local government, of the regional medical programs and of *consumers* of health services. A majority of the members of such councils are to be representatives of consumers.

Administration
Health Resources Administration (Comprehensive Health Planning Service)

17. HEALTH MANPOWER LEGISLATION UNDER THE PUBLIC HEALTH SERVICE ACT

The first federal legislation particularly addressed to the question of health manpower, except for certain temporary wartime programs, was the *Health Amendments Act of 1956.* This law authorized under Title III of the Public Health Service Act traineeships for professional public health personnel[87] and for advanced training of professional nurses. A third provision amended the Vocational Education Act of 1946 to authorize grants for programs for practical nurse training.[88]

A program of formula grants to *schools of public health* was established in 1958. (PL 85-544).[89] In 1960 there was added (PL 86-720) a program of project grants to schools of public health and schools of nursing or engineering providing graduate or specialized public health training. The *Graduate Public Health Training Amendments of 1964* broadened eligibility for project grants to include other institutions providing such training.

---

[87]Physicians, engineers, nurses and other professional health personnel.

[88]Such training had been permitted under the general vocational education program, but this amendment made specific provisions for this.

[89]By earmarking for this purpose a portion of the funds authorized to the states for public health services. In 1966 (PL 89-749) the program was separately provided for.

Health Professions Educational
Assistance Act of 1963

This Act inaugurated, under Title VII of the Public Health Service Act, the program of *construction grants* for teaching facilities: grants for the construction or rehabilitation of facilities for training of physicians, dentists, pharmacists, podiatrists, nurses,[90] or professional public health personnel, these contigent on increased first year enrollments. Also authorized was a program of *student loan funds* at schools of medicine, osteopathy, and dentistry.[91]

Nurse Training Act of 1964

This Act added Title VIII, "Nurse Training," to the Public Health Service Act. This authorized separate funding for construction grants for schools of nursing and extended eligibility to associate degree and diploma schools, these were also contingent on increased enrollment. Also authorized were project grants to the schools to improve and expand their training programs, and formula grants to diploma schools.[92] Provision was also made for the establishment of *student loan funds* at schools of nursing.

Health Professions Assistance
Amendments of 1965

These amendments authorized a program of grants to "improve the quality of schools of medicine, dentistry, osteopathy, optometry and podiatry." These were *basic improvement* (institutional) grants related to enrollment and contingent on increased enrollment, and *special improvement* grants. *Scholarship* grants were also authorized for these schools, plus schools of pharmacy. The student loan program was expanded, with provisions for partial cancellation for physicians, dentists, and optometrists practicing in shortage areas, and eligibility was extended to students of pharmacy and podiatry.

Allied Health Professions Personnel
Training Act of 1966

This Act established programs of *construction* and *improvement grants* for training centers for allied health professions,[93] generally patterned after those in the previous legislation. For the construction grants, the facilitation of training in *three or more related* (of specified) curriculums was to be

---

[90] In schools with baccalaureate or graduate degree programs.

[91] Following the general pattern of loan funds established under the National Defense Education Act of 1958. Students of optometry and veterinary medicine were subsequently included (PL 88-654, 89-709).

[92] Formula grants related to the number of "federally sponsored" students (those receiving loans from the fund also established), and to increased enrollment.

[93] Defined as a "junior college, college, or university which provides education leading to a baccalaureate or associate degree (or equivalents) or a higher degree in medical technology, dental hygiene, or other curriculums specified by regulations. . . ."

taken into account. *Advanced traineeships* for allied health professions personnel were authorized, as were project grants related to the training of new types of health technologists. Additional loan cancellation was provided for physicians, dentists, and optometrists practicing in poor rural areas. Revolving funds for loans to student loan funds were authorized under Titles VII and VIII and the latter title was further amended to authorize "opportunity grants for nursing education" (*scholarships* for nursing students of exceptional financial need), and contracts with agencies and institutions to identify such individuals and to publicize sources of financial aid.

Health Manpower Act of 1968

This Act extended, with some changes, most of the previous programs. Among the changes were the extension of the institutional and special project grants to schools of pharmacy and veterinary medicine and the addition of students of veterinary medicine to the scholarship program.[94] Also, the Secretary was directed to prepare a report on Title VII programs.

Health Training Improvement
Act of 1970

This Act provided for institutional grants for new schools of health professions and directed the Secretary to report to Congress on the need for emergency financial assistance to medical and dental schools. It extended, with some changes, the grant programs for allied health professions. Changes included broadening of eligibility for advanced traineeships to other organizations and institutions in addition to those defined as training centers. Authorization was added for *special project* grants and contracts related to training or retraining of allied health personnel. Also authorized was a program of grants and contracts for projects related to encouraging and assisting the entry into allied health professions training of individuals of financial, educational, or cultural need, and provision was made for grants for *scholarships, work-study programs,* and *student loan funds.* The Secretary was directed to conduct a study of the provisions and programs relating to allied health professions in the Public Health Service Act and other Acts, and also to report on the major problems associated with licensure, certification, and other qualifications for health personnel.

Comprehensive Health Manpower Training
Act of 1971[95]

This Act extended the program of construction grants for health research and teaching facilities, raised the latter grant ceiling to 70-80 percent,

---

[94]These schools had become eligible for construction grants in 1966 (PL 89-709).

[95]This is a particularly complex and important piece of legislation. Those with particular interest in the subject would be well advised to read the complete law and the

and mandated an opportunity for review and comment by the appropriate 314a and 314b agencies. Provisions for construction loan guarantees and interest subsidies were added.

The previous institutional grants were replaced by a new system of *capitation grants* for each student enrolled in health professional schools, again contingent upon increased first-year enrollment and upon submission of plans for projects for improvement of teaching programs in at least three of nine specified categories.[96] *Start up* assistance to new schools of medicine, osteopathy, and dentistry was authorized, also in the form of capitation grants.

Special project grants to health professions schools were authorized for a wide variety of activities related to professional education in priority areas and the utilization of health personnel; *contracts* were authorized with other health and educational entities for similar projects. Additionally, grants were authorized to schools in *financial distress.*

A new program of grants and contracts, *health manpower education initiative awards,* was authorized for health and educational entities to support a wide variety of projects for the purpose of "improving the distribution, supply, quality, utilization, and efficiency of health personnel and the health services delivery system;" these awards are to be coordinated with the area's regional medical program. Additional grants were authorized for special projects related to enrollment of students who might be expected to practice in shortage areas, and students who are financially or otherwise disadvantaged.

The *loan* provisions were broadened to provide up to 85 percent cancellation for health professionals practicing for three years in shortage areas. *Scholarships* for needy students were increased and provision was made for the total amounts available for the scholarship funds to be increased according to numbers of students enrolled from low income backgrounds. A new *physician shortage area* scholarship program was established for medical students who agree to practice *primary care* (one year for each scholarship year) in an area of physician shortage or with substantial numbers of migratory agricultural workers.

Another new program included grants for training, traineeships, and fellowships in family medicine; annual capitation grants for approved graduate training programs for physicians and dentists in primary care and other designated

---

House Committee report.

An extensive description and commentary on this and other recent health manpower legislation is found in *Federal Laws: Health/Environment Manpower,* by John T. Grupenhoff and Stephen P. Strickland (Washington, D.C.: Science and Communication Group, 1972).

[96]These covered such activities as curriculum improvements (including shortening), interdisciplinary training, training for new roles or types of personnel (including physician assistants and nurse practitioners), teaching of health care organization; training in clinical pharmacology, nutrition, and management of drug and alcohol abuse, programs related to admission and retention of disadvantaged students, and projects related to training primary care health professionals and family medicine.

shortage areas of care; grants for advanced training, traineeships and fellowships for health professions teaching personnel; and grants related to the use of computer technology in health care.

Finally, there were a number of miscellaneous provisions relating to health manpower. A National Health Manpower Clearinghouse was established. The Secretary was directed to "use his best efforts to provide, to each county certified by him to be without the services of a physician . . . at least one physician in the Public Health Service. . . ."[97] The Comptroller General was directed to conduct a study of *health facilities construction costs.* The Secretary was directed to arrange for a study (preferably by the National Academy of Sciences) of the annual per student *educational cost* of schools of health professions (including nursing) and to prepare a report on the parts of Title VII related to health professionals education.

Nurse Training Act of 1971[98]

This Act extended the construction grant program, increased the grant ceiling to 67-75 percent, and added provisions for loan construction guarantees and interest subsidies. The program of special project grants was broadened to cover a wide variety of activities related to nursing and interdisciplinary training; contract authorization was added, and provision was made for grants to schools in *financial distress.*

The program of formula grants to diploma schools[99] was replaced by annual *capitation* grants for nursing schools, contingent on increased enrollment,[100] with additional amounts authorized for further enrollment increase, and for schools with training programs for nurse midwives, family health nurses, and other nurse practitioners. An additional requirement for these grants was that a school submit a plan to carry out projects in at least three of several categories related to improved nursing training, and the Secretary was directed to report to the appropriate Congressional committees on the carrying out of these projects. A separate program of *start up* grants was authorized for new nurse training programs.

The advanced traineeships and the student loan program were continued, with provision made for loan cancellation up to 85 percent after five years of full-time nursing employment, and, for practice in an area of shortage, up to 85 percent after three years. *Half-time* students were also made eligible for loans. The *scholarship* program was extended and expanded, with half-time students becoming eligible.

---

[97]Amending the Emergency Health Personnel Act (National Health Service Corps).

[98]This is the companion to the Comprehensive Health Manpower Act and contains many analogous provisions.

[99]This program was not actually funded and thus was never implemented.

[100]Which could be waived if circumstances warranted.

Additionally, grants and contracts were authorized to health or educational entities for activities related to the enrollment in schools of nursing of persons such as veterans with health field experience, the financially and otherwise disadvantaged, and licensed practical nurses. Finally, the Secretary was directed to report to Congress on the administration and impact of the Title VIII programs.

Administration
Health Resources Administration (Bureau of Health Resources Development)

Advisory Councils
National Advisory Council on Health Professions Education
National Advisory Council on Nurse Training

Note
A large number of grant programs are authorized in this legislation. It should be kept in mind that the actual receipt of grants is dependent upon the level of funds actually appropriated by Congress, and the allocation of funds by the administrative agencies. The continuation of many of the programs has also, as of this writing, become problematical due to differing and changing views of health manpower training priorities in the Executive and Legislative branches.

18. HEALTH MAINTENANCE ORGANIZATION ACT OF 1973

An Act to amend the Public Health Service Act to provide assistance and encouragement for the establishment and expansion of health maintenance organizations, and for other purposes.

A new title, XIII, *Health Maintenance Organizations,* is added to the Public Health Service Act.

Summary of Major Provisions

Financial Assistance for the Development of Health Maintenance Organizations
There is established a program of financial assistance for the development or expansion of health maintenance organizations. This comprises

1. Grants and contracts to determine the feasibility of development or expansion of individual health maintenance organizations;
2. Grants and contracts for planning projects;
3. Grants, contracts and loan guarantees for initial development;
4. Loans and loan guarantees for initial operating costs (to offset, when necessary, losses during the first 36 months.)

For purposes of this title, a health maintenance organization is a legal entity which provides basic and supplemental services to its members, and is organized and operated in a prescribed manner.

Basic medical services are to be provided for a set, periodic payment fixed under a community rating system. These services are:

1. Physician services
2. Inpatient and outpatient services
3. Medically necessary emergency health services
4. Short-term outpatient evaluative and crisis intervention mental health services (not over 20 visits)
5. Medical treatment and referral services for alcohol and drug abuse
6. Laboratory and X-ray services
7. Home health services
8. Preventive services (including voluntary family planning and infertility services, and preventive dental care and eye examinations for children)

Nominal additional payments may be required for specific basic services.

The basic health services payment may be supplemented by nominal charges for specific services (copayment) unless this is determined to be an undue barrier to the delivery of health services.

Supplemental health services are to be made available to enrolled members who wish to contract for them. These are:

1. Intermediate and long-term care
2. Vision care and dental and mental health services not included under basic services
3. Provision of prescription drugs

At least 20 percent of the appropriated funds are to be allocated to rural health maintenance organizations.

Professional services which are provided as basic services are in general to be provided through health professionals who are members of the staff of the health maintenance organizations or through medical groups or individual practice associations.

The requirements for a health maintenance organization include

1. Evidence of fiscal responsibility
2. Enrollment of persons broadly representative of the age, social and income groups within the area served; except that not more than 75 percent of the members may be enrolled from a medically underserved population, unless the area served is a rural area

3. A policy making board, at least one-third of whose membership are (enrolled) members of the organization, and with equitable representation of the medically underserved population
4. Arrangements for a quality assurance program
5. Provision of medical social services and health education services
6. Provision for continuing education for its health professional staff

Organizations serving Medicare and Medicaid beneficiaries are not required to provide basic services which are not compensated under these programs, nor to fix payments by community rating.

Employees Health Benefit Plans

Every employer of 25 or more persons is to include in health benefit plans offered to employees the option to enroll in health maintenance organizations which are providing services in the areas in which the employees reside.

Restrictive State Laws and Practices

State requirements which prevent an entity from functioning as a health maintenance organization (as defined in this legislation) shall not apply. Specifically, preempted restrictions are:

1. Requirement of approval by a medical society of services furnished
2. Requirement that physicians constitute all or a percentage of the governing body
3. Requirement that all or a percentage of physicians be permitted to participate in the provision of services
4. Certain requirements for insurers
5. Prohibition of solicitation of members through advertising of services, charges or other nonprofessional aspects of an organization's operation

Quality Assurance

A new part is added to Title III of the Public Health Service Act: Part K—*Quality Assurance.*

The Secretary, through the Assistant Secretary of Health, is to conduct research and evaluation programs respecting the effectiveness, administration and enforcement of quality assurance programs.

The Secretary is also directed to make an annual report to Congress and the President on the quality of health care in the United States, the operation of quality assurance programs, and advances made through research and evaluation.

Other Studies and Reports

The Secretary is to contract with a nonprofit organization of recognized competence for the conduct of a general study in the area of quality assurance. The study is to include analysis of methodologies, the delineation of basic principles for quality assurance systems, the definition of need in the area of research and evaluation related to health care quality, and the provision of methods for quality assessment from the point of view of consumers. Interim and final reports of the study are to be submitted to the appropriate Congressional committees.

19. SUMMARY OF PUBLIC HEALTH
SERVICE ACT TITLES

Title I.   Short Title and Definitions

Title II.   Administration

        General Organization of the Public Health Service and the Commissioned Corps.

Title III.   General Powers and Duties of the Public Health Service

     A. Research and Investigation

        Includes National Health Surveys and Studies, Public Health Traineeships and Project Grants, and Health Services for Agricultural Migrants

     B. Federal-State Cooperation

        Includes Comprehensive Health Planning and Public Health Services (Section 314).

     C. Hospitals, Medical Examinations and Medical Care

     D. Lepers

     E. Narcotic Addicts and Other Drug Abuses

     F. Licensing—Biological Products and Clinical Laboratories and Control of Radiation

     G. Quarantine and Inspection

     H. Grants to Alaska for Mental Health (Repealed)

     I. National Library of Medicine

     J. Assistance to Medical Libraries

     K. Quality Assurance

Title IV.   National Research Institutes

     A. National Cancer Institute

     B. National Heart Institute

     C. National Institute of Dental Research

     D. National Institute on Arthritis, Metabolism and Digestive Diseases; National Institute of Neurological Diseases and Stroke; and Other Institutes

     E. National Institutes of Child Health and Human Development and of General Medical Sciences

     F. National Eye Institute

Title V.   Miscellaneous

Title VI.   Assistance for Construction and Modernization of Hospitals and Other Medical Facilities
   A. Grants and Loans for Construction and Modernization of Hospitals and Other Medical Facilities
   B. Loan Guarantees and Loans for Modernization and Construction of Hospitals and Other Medical Facilities
   C. Construction or Modernization of Emergency Rooms
   D. General

Title VII. Health Research and Teaching Facilities and Training of Professional Health Personnel
   A. Grants for Construction of Health Research Facilities
   B. Grants for Construction of Teaching Facilities for Medical, Dental and Other Health Personnel
   C. Student Loans
   D. Grants for Family Medicine, Training, Traineeships, and Fellowships and Computer Technology Health Care Demonstration Programs
   E. Grants and Contracts to Improve the Quality of Schools of Medicine, Osteopathy, Dentistry, Veterinary Medicine, Optometry, Pharmacy and Podiatry; Health Manpower Educational Initiative Awards
   F. Scholarship Grants to Schools of Medicine, Osteopathy, Dentistry, Optometry, Podiatry, Pharmacy, or Veterinary Medicine
   G. Training in the Allied Health Professions
   H. General Provisions

Title VIII. Nurse Training
   A. Grants for Expansion and Improvement of Nurse Training
   B. Assistance to Nursing Students
   C. General (National Advisory Council on Nurse Training; Review Committee)
   D. Scholarship Grants to Schools of Nursing

Title IX.   Education, Research, Training, and Demonstrations in the Fields of Heart Disease, Cancer, Stroke, Kidney Disease, and Other Related Diseases

Title X.   Population Research and Voluntary Family Planning Programs

Title XI.   Genetic Blood Disorders
   A. Sickle Cell Anemia Programs
   B. Cooley's Anemia Programs

Title XII. Emergency Medical Services Systems

Title XIII. Health Maintenance Organizations

20. MENTAL RETARDATION FACILITIES AND COMMUNITY MENTAL HEALTH CENTERS CONSTRUCTION ACT OF 1963

> An Act to provide assistance in combating mental retardation through grants for construction of research centers and grants for facilities for the mentally retarded and assistance in improving mental health through grants for construction of community mental health centers, and for other purposes.

Background

Congressional interest in the problem of mental health was first expressed in the *Mental Health Act of 1946* which specifically provided for the inclusion of mental health problems in the grant-in-aid programs of the Public Health Service Act and established the National Institute of Mental Health patterned after the National Cancer Institute. The *Mental Health Study Act of 1955* authorized grants to facilitate a program of research into resources and methods for care of the mentally ill,[101] and in 1956 the *Health Amendments Act* added special project grants particularly directed to the problems of state mental hospitals. Legislation addressed to the problem of mental retardation was added in 1963 in the *Maternal and Child Health and Mental Retardation Planning Amendments.*[102]

Summary of Major Provisions

Title I. Construction of Research Centers and Facilities for the Mentally Retarded—"Mental Retardation Facilities Construction Act"

Part A. Grants for Construction of Centers for Research on Mental Retardation and Related Aspects of Human Development

Amends Title VII of the Public Health Service Act to authorize grants to assist in the construction of facilities for research relating to mental retardation.[103] Federal participation: up to 75 percent.

Part B. Project Grants for Construction of University Affiliated Facilities for the Mentally Retarded

Grants for the construction of university-affiliated facilities providing a full range of inpatient and outpatient services; for demonstrating specialized

---

[101] The resultant Joint Commission on Mental Illness and Health published a final report, *Action for Mental Health,* in 1961.

[102] See p. 125

[103] Under the program of construction grants established by the Health Research Facilities Act of 1956.

services for the mentally retarded; or for clinical training of physicians and other specialized personnel. Federal participation: up to 75 percent.

Part C.   Grants for the Construction of Facilities for the Mentally Retarded

Grants to the states for the construction of community facilities for the mentally retarded; patterned after the Hill-Burton program. Federal share: 33 1/3 to 66 2/3 percent.

Title II.   Construction of Community Mental Health Centers– "Community Mental Health Centers Act"

Grants to the states for construction of community mental health centers, also generally patterned after the Hill-Burton program. Federal share: 33 1/3 to 66 2/3 percent.

Title III.   Training of Teachers of Mentally Retarded and Other Handicapped Children

Extends and strengthens existing programs for training teachers of mentally retarded and deaf children,[104] and expands them to include the training of teachers of other handicapped children.

Title IV.   General

Definitions include:

Community Mental Health Center–A facility providing services for the prevention or diagnosis of mental illness, or care and treatment of mentally ill patients, or rehabilitation of such persons, which services are provided principally for persons residing in a particular community or communities in or near which the facility is situated.

Construction–Construction of new buildings, expansion, remodeling and alteration of existing buildings, and initial equipment for any such buildings.

Amendments to the Mental Retardation and Community Mental Health Centers Legislation

The 1965 amendments to this legislation included provisions for grants to assist in meeting the initial cost of professional and technical personnel for community mental health centers (30-75 percent), and grants to institutions of higher education for construction of facilities for research in the field of education of handicapped children.

---

[104] Legislation (PL 85-929, 1958) authorizing grants to educational institutions and agencies for training teachers of mentally retarded children.

The Mental Health Amendments of 1967 extended the program of grants for construction and initial staffing of community mental health centers and amended the term "construction" to include acquisition of existing buildings. The Mental Retardation Amendments of 1967 extended the program of construction grants for university affiliated and community facilities for the mentally retarded, and established a program of initial staffing grants analogous to those for community mental health centers. A new title was added: Title V—"Training of Physical Educators and Recreation Personnel for Mentally Retarded and Other Handicapped Children." This authorized grants to educational institutions for the training of such personnel and for related research and demonstration projects.

The Alcoholic and Narcotic Addict Rehabilitation Amendments of 1968[105] added new provisions to the Community Mental Health Centers Act, relating to alcoholism and narcotic addiction: grants for construction and initial staffing of facilities for the treatment and rehabilitation of alcoholics[106] and narcotic addicts and grants for special training programs and evaluation studies relating to narcotic addiciton services.

The Community Mental Health Centers Amendments of 1970 extended the program of construction grants and changed the definition of construction to include the acquisition of land. The duration of initial staffing grants was lengthened to eight years and, for centers in poverty areas, the grant ceiling was increased to 70-90 percent. Provision was also made for centers in poverty areas to begin operation (for 18 months) without furnishing all the "essential" components of comprehensive mental health services.[107] Additionally, grants were authorized to local agencies for development of community mental health services in rural or urban poverty areas.

The program of grants for facilities and services for alcoholics and narcotic addicts was also extended,[108] the duration of the staffing grants lengthened, and the grant ceiling increased, for centers in poverty areas. Special project grants were authorized for training, surveys, treatment and rehabilitation projects.

The Community Mental Health Centers Act was further amended by the addition of a part on Mental Health of Children. This authorized grants

---

[105] A section of the Public Health Service Amendments of 1968 which also amended the Regional Medical Programs and the Hill-Burton and Migratory Workers Programs.

[106] These facilities to be associated with other mental health services program, including community mental health centers.

[107] As specified in regulations, these services are:
"1. Inpatient services
2. Outpatient services
3. Partial hospitalization services—must include at least day care service
4. Emergency services provided 24 hours per day . . .
5. Consultation and education services [for] community agencies and professional personnel."

[108] The alcoholism section of this program had not yet been implemented.

for construction of facilities[109] for the mental health of children, the cost of professional and technical personnel for new facilities or new services, and for training and program evaluation.

The *Comprehensive Drug Abuse Prevention and Control Act of 1970*[110] included provisions broadening the scope of narcotic addiction programs to include drug abuse and drug dependence, authorized grants for programs and activities related to drug education and special project grants for drug abuse and addiction treatment and rehabilitation.

The Developmental Disabilities Services and Facilities Construction Amendments of 1970 extended the mental retardation programs and broadened the language of the legislation to include other neurological handicapping conditions.

Provisions of the *Comprehensive Alcohol Abuse and Alcoholism Prevention, Treatment and Rehabilitation Act of 1970* added to the Community Mental Health Centers Act provisions for project grants and contracts in the area of prevention and treatment of alcohol abuse and alcoholism.[111]

21. SUMMARY OF MENTAL RETARDATION AND MENTAL HEALTH CENTER TITLES

Title I. Services and Facilities for the Mentally Retarded and Persons with Other Developmental Disabilities
   A. Construction of Research Facilities (Expired)
   B. Construction, Demonstration, and Training Grants for University-Affiliated Facilities for Persons with Developmental Disabilities
   C. Grants for Planning, Provision of Services, and Construction and Operation of Facilities for Persons with Developmental Disabilities
   D. Grants for the Cost of Professional and Technical Personnel of Community Mental Retardation Facilities

Title II. Community Mental Health Centers
   A. Grants for Construction
   B. Grants for Initial Cost of Professional and Technical Personnel of Centers
   C. Alcoholism

---

[109] Associated with a community mental health center or other appropriate facility.

[110] Title II of this legislation is named the *Controlled Substances Act.* It contains provisions for drug abuse related control and enforcement by the Department of Justice.

[111] This comprehensive alcoholism act also (1) established the National Institute on Alcohol Abuse and Alcoholism in the National Institute of Mental Health and a national Advisory Council on Alcohol Abuse and Alcoholism, (2) directed the Civil Service Commission to develop appropriate prevention, treatment, and rehabilitation programs for Federal employees, and (3) authorized formula grants to the states for projects related to prevention, treatment and rehabilitation.

D. Narcotic Addiction, Drug Abuse, and Drug Dependence Prevention and Rehabilitation

E. General Provisions

F. Mental Health of Children

Title III.   Training of Teachers of Mentally Retarded and Other Handicapped Children

Title IV.   General (definitions and general provisions)

Title V.   Training of Physical Educators and Recreation Personnel for Mentally Retarded and Other Handicapped Children

22. ECONOMIC OPPORTUNITY ACT OF 1964— "ANTI-POVERTY PROGRAM"

An Act to mobilize the human and financial resources of the Nation to combat poverty in the United States.

Title I.   Work Training and Work Study Programs

A. Establishes the Job Corps (conservation camps and residential training centers).

B. Work-training programs for unemployed youths and young adults (Neighborhood Youth Corps).

C. Work-study programs in colleges and universities for students from low income families

Title II.   Urban and Rural Community Action Programs

A. Grants for antipoverty programs to be planned and carried out at the community level. Programs are to be administered by the communities and are to mobilize all available resources and facilities in a coordinated attack on poverty.

B. Grants to the states for basic adult education programs.

C. Voluntary assistance program for needy children (information and coordination office).

Title III.   Antipoverty Programs in Rural Areas

A. Loans to low income rural families.

B. Assistance for housing, sanitation, education, and child care programs for migrant farm workers.

C. Indemnity payments to farmers for pesticide-contaminated milk.

Title IV.   Assistance to Small Business Concerns

Loans and management training for small businesses.

Title V.   Work Experience Programs

Grants for experimental and demonstration work experience and training programs for unemployed persons on public assistance.

Title VI.   Administration and Coordination

Establishes the Office of Economic Opportunity and provides for administration of the Act. Authorizes the program *Volunteers in Service to America* (VISTA).

Title VII.   Exemption of Income for Public Assistance Purposes
                  Exemption of part or all of earnings under the Economic Oppor-
                  tunity Act from consideration as income or resources of public
                  assistance recipients.

Office of Economic Opportunity
(Executive Office of the President)

1. Direct responsibility for the *Job Corps, community action programs, VISTA,*
    and the programs for migrant farm workers;
2. Indirect (delegated) responsibility for the work study, adult education and
    work experience programs (HEW); the work training programs (Department
    of Labor); the special rural programs (Department of Agriculture); and the
    small business programs (Small Business Administration);
3. Coordination of the poverty-related programs of all federal agencies.

Community Action Programs

The legislation defines a community action program eligible for
federal assistance as one which:

> Mobilizes and utilizes resources, public or private . . . in an attack
> on poverty;
>
> Provides services, assistance and other activities [which] give prom-
> ise of progress toward the elimination of poverty or a cause or
> causes of poverty . . . ;
>
> Is developed, conducted and administered with the *maximum feasi-
> ble participation of residents of the areas and members of the groups
> served*; and
>
> Is conducted, administered or coordinated by a public or nonprofit
> agency, or combination thereof.

Community action programs could be conducted in such fields as
employment, job training and counseling, health, vocational rehabilitation,
housing, home management, welfare, and special remedial and other noncurricular
educational assistance.

Among the many programs which have been developed under the
community action provisions, and which have been given statutory recognition
in amendments to this Title, are the OEO neighborhood health centers (comprehensive health services programs), the Head Start child development programs,
the legal services programs and the family planning and drug rehabilitation programs.

The Economic Opportunity Act, often controversial, has been much
amended, and many administrative changes have been made. Notably, the Job

Corps and Neighborhood Youth Corps are now administered by the Department of Labor, the VISTA program has been combined with the Peace Corps in a new ACTION agency, the Head Start program has been placed in HEW's Office of Child Development, and many of the neighborhood health centers have been transferred to the Public Health Service. As of this writing, the future of the Office of Economic Opportunity and its remaining community action programs is uncertain.

A NOTE TO THE READER

Many details of the book will be altered by the swift pace of changing events.

This is particularly true of these sections dealing with federal legislation and the organization of federal agencies.

In the case of Congressional activity this problem can be dealt with without undue difficulty if the interested reader will, once having acquired a basic understanding of the progression of the laws, develop a systematic approach to keeping abreast of developments. One method would be the regular scanning of the *Congressional Quarterly* or the *U.S. Code and Administrative News.* Systematic review of one of the many Washington newsletters would also be useful. Examples of these are the *Washington Report on Medicine and Health* and the letters published by the various interested associations, such as the American Public Health Association, the American Public Welfare Association, and the Association of American Medical Colleges. A regular *Memorandum* published by the Special Committee on Aging, United States Senate, is good for matters affecting the elderly, including Social Security amendments.

I have yet to find a really good way to keep up with the various activities and reorganizations of the federal agencies. The above newsletters are helpful. Direct inquiries to the agency of interest will elicit information, although the substantive quality varies widely. Some put out regular newsletters.

Significant reorganizations and all administrative regulations are published in the *Federal Register.* Those who are involved with federal programs usually take care to watch for these.

Obtaining Documents

Single copies of bills, laws, committee hearings and reports can usually be obtained from the House or Senate Document Room, Washington, D.C.; zip codes 20515 and 20510, respectively. (Enclose a self-addressed label.) These can often also be obtained from the Congressional Committees or from individual Congressmen and Senators.

Similarly, single copies of many reports and publications can be obtained from the relevant agencies.

The U.S. Government Printing Office publishes a monthly catalog of published documents, which are for sale at a usually nominal price.

References

Congressional Quarterly and Almanac, (Washington, D.C.: Congressional Quarterly, Inc.) Weekly and yearly summary and commentary on Congressional activities.

U.S. Code Congressional and Administrative News, (St. Paul, Minnesota: West Publishing Co.) Monthly and yearly Congressional summary with texts of newly passed laws and related committee reports.

Washington Report on Medicine and Health, (Washington, D.C.: McGraw-Hill, Inc.) A weekly commentary on federal events.

Chapter Five

State and Local Health Activities

In general, the responsibility for the general public health and welfare resides with the states.[1]

The many state activities related to health include:

1. Traditional public health functions related to the promotion of health and the prevention of disease, such as communicable disease control, sanitation and the assurance of the quality of water and food supplies.
2. Provision of direct institutional services for long-term conditions such as tuberculosis, mental illness, mental retardation, and chronic disease. Such services are generally beyond the capacity of the private or public sectors of the local communities.
3. Regulatory Functions. These include the licensing of health professionals and of health facilities; the regulation, under the insurance laws, of health insurance companies and organizations; and the establishment of health and safety codes for housing, institutions and industry. A recent development has been the enactment, in many states, of "certificate of need" legislation controlling the construction and establishment of health facilities and programs.
4. Planning Functions. The states participate in health planning activities through state and local comprehensive health planning agencies.
5. Educational Functions. There are many programs for health manpower education and training in the state colleges, universities, and other institutions. These include medicine, nursing, pharmacy, and many others.

---

[1] In theory, all governmental authority resides in the states, except as delegated by them to the federal government, under the Constitution or to local jurisdictions, by legislation.

179

6. Administration of federally aided programs. Most federal grant-in-aid programs are administered by the cooperating state agencies. (Examples are the Hill-Burton, Medicaid, community mental health centers, and vocational rehabilitation programs.) Certain aspects of other programs are also handled by state agencies; (for example, the surveying and certification of institutional providers of services under Medicare).

Health-related services in the states, and as delegated to the counties, cities, and towns, are provided by a complex and ever-changing variety of agencies and organizations in patterns which differ from state to state. Many of them are lodged in *departments of public health*. Many are typically lodged elsewhere. For example, there is often a separate state department of mental health; licensing of health manpower may be a responsibility of departments of education; vocational rehabilitation programs are often administered by separate agencies; occupational health (industrial hygiene) is usually lodged in state departments of labor; and school health is commonly 'the responsibility of boards of education. Recently, several states have placed environmental control programs in separate agencies.

Public Health Departments

The traditional "basic six"[2] functions of public health agencies are:

1. Collection of *vital statistics* of births, deaths, and reportable diseases
2. Control of communicable diseases,[3] including tuberculosis and venereal diseases
3. Environmental sanitation, including water quality and supervision of foods and eating places
4. Public health laboratory services
5. Maternal and child health, including school health
6. Health education

Notable additions to the list in recent years have been activities directed to problems such as *nutrition, chronic disease, dental health, radiological control, air quality control, alcohol and drug abuse* and *family planning.*

Health agencies, at various levels, have traditionally been organized in appropriate divisions and bureaus to carry out these functions which are largely concerned with the prevention of disease and disability.

In recent years there has been a great increase in health planning, regulatory, standard-setting, and monitoring functions, especially with regard to health care institutions such as hospitals and nursing homes. These activities

---

[2]As set forth in the report *Local Health Units for the Nation* by Haven Emerson, M.D., The Commonwealth Fund, 1945.

[3]Public health had its beginnings in efforts by society to control the spread of disease.

were originally greatly stimulated by the federal Hill-Burton legislation directed to hospital planning and construction and more recently by provision of the Medicare-Medicaid and Comprehensive Health Planning laws. These trends have been augmented by the rapid development of "certificate of need" legislation by the states. Many of these functions have been placed in health agencies but many have been placed in other agencies, the pattern again varying from state to state.

Many health departments have also become increasingly concerned with the problems of the provision of direct medical care services, especially to low income populations.

State Health Departments

In most of the states, primary responsibility for public health is lodged in a separate state department of health.[4] There is also usually a *Board of Health,* with varying advisory, policy and administrative functions, with members generally appointed by the governor. The chief executive officer (health officer, director, commissioner) is also usually appointed by the governor or by the board.

State departments of health delegate most direct services to the local departments[5] providing them general liaison, consultation, and special services as needed. The state agencies usually retain certain statewide regulatory and planning functions, such as professional and health facilities licensure, Hill-Burton administration and statewide comprehensive health planning.[6]

Local Health Departments

With a few exceptions, mostly in some rural western counties,[7] all areas of the United States are served by local health units—county, city, town, or (a few instances) combined city and county.[8] The number and scope of services provided vary greatly.

There are local *boards of health* with members appointed by elected officials—county commissioners or supervisors, mayors, or town selectmen. The health officer is typically appointed by the board generally in accordance with qualifications set by the state department of health.[9]

---

[4] In some states, the health agency is combined with one or more other agencies, most often the department of public welfare (now commonly termed "Social Services").

[5] A notable exception being the operation of such facilities as chronic disease and tuberculosis hospitals.

[6] The state comprehensive health planning "A" agencies are variously lodged in state health departments, in interdepartmental commissions, or in governors' executive offices.

[7] But also in parts of New York State and all of Rhode Island.

[8] Where there is no local health unit, services are provided by regional or district offices of the state health department.

[9] Generally, though not invariably, the health officer is a physician.

Staff of a local health unit will include as a minimum the health officer, one or more public health nurses, and one or more sanitary engineers or sanitarians. With increasing scope of responsibilities, the number and types of professional and technical staff will increase commensurately and may include dentists, social workers, health educators, nutritionists, epidemiologists, special laboratory personnel, and many others.

Where many and complex services are provided, the health officer will serve as director or commissioner of an organized department of health with appropriate divisions; here the basic unit for provision of direct services to the population is usually the *health center*. Large health departments may be partially decentralized, with district health officers and centers.

The health center will house services such as maternity and family planning clinics, well baby and child health clinics, tuberculosis and venereal disease units, dental clinics (usually for children), nutrition and health educative services, and field personnel for environmental health programs. Some health centers in low income communities have in recent years been providing treatment as well as preventive services for children, usually in cooperation with a local hospital; health centers have also been the base for some of the federally funded health care programs and neighborhood health centers.

"Umbrella Agencies"

In recent years a number of state and local jurisdictions have attempted to consolidate and streamline health and welfare services by combining related departments and agencies into one overall administrative structure. These "umbrella agencies" or "super agencies" have involved varying combinations of departments of health, hospitals,[10] mental health, public welfare, rehabilitation, youth services, and others. Examples of such amalgamations are the North Carolina Department of Human Resources, the Suffolk County (New York) Department of Health Services, and the New York City Health Services Administration.

Reference

John J. Hanlon, *Principles of Public Health Administration,* Fifth Edition (Saint Louis: The C.V Mosby Company, 1969).

---

[10] In some jurisdictions which maintain county or municipal hospitals.

Chapter Six

Ambulatory Care (Non-Institutional Care)

Strictly speaking, the term *ambulatory care* refers to care rendered to patients who come to physicians' offices, outpatient departments, and health centers. However, it often includes by extension other hospital-related, non-inpatient components of care such as emergency and home care services. The term is also often used with the same connotation as *community medicine.*

This field is complex and many of its aspects are rapidly changing in concept and terminology. The following are brief descriptions of components which are of particular importance or current interest.

Forms of Physician Practice

Solo Practice.[1] Independent practice by a physician usually using his own facilities and equipment, but sometimes sharing these with one or more other physicians. A formal arrangement for using common facilities is often termed an *association.*

Partnership. A legal agreement between two or more physicians to share income and assets in an unincorporated business, with each partner legally the agent of the other. Many group practices are in fact partnerships, although they frequently include salaried physicians among their staff.

Group Practice. There is no one generally accepted definition of group practice, but the common denominator is a voluntary association of three or more physicians in medical practice who use common facilities and share income in a designated way.

The American Medical Association defines a group practice as "the application of medical services by three or more physicians formally organized to provide medical care, consultation, diagnosis and/or treatment

---

[1]Legally, a solo practitioner is a *sole proprietor*—a one-man owner of an unincorporated business.

through the joint use of equipment and personnel, and with the income from medical practice distributed in accordance with methods previously determined by members of the group."

Groups so defined consist of three categories:

1. Single specialty groups
2. General practice groups
3. Multi-specialty groups (providing services in at least two specialties)

Other definitions specify that services include those of more than one specialty.

The first group practice, a multispecialty group, was the well-known Mayo Clinic, established in Rochester, Minnesota in the decade prior to 1900. Group practices began to develop in significant numbers in the 1920s, particularly in the West and Midwest, but their growth was relatively slow, with further relative increases after World War II. In 1969 there were upward of 6,000 group practices, involving about 40,000 physicians. Of these, about half were single specialty groups.[2]

Many of the larger group practices are associated with pre-payment plans; among these are the Permanente groups (Kaiser Foundation Health Plan) and the HIP groups (Health Insurance Plans of Greater New York, New York City).

Associations
American Association of Medical Clinics
Medical Group Management Association (formerly National Association of Clinic Managers)

Professional Corporation
A legal entity which is distinct from its members. There is limited liability for corporate debts, but a physician member remains liable for his own negligent acts. Most states now permit the establishment of professional corporations, which carry certain tax advantages and other benefits. Solo practitioners as well as groups of physicians may incorporate.[3]

Centers, Programs and Agencies

Outpatient Department. In the past often termed "dispensary,"[4] now apt to be called an ambulatory care service. A hospital department where

---

[2]For an extensive survey of groups, see: C. Todd and M. E. McNamara, *Medical Groups in the U.S. 1969*, Special Statistical Series, American Medical Association, 1971.

[3]A series of court decisions led the Internal Revenue Service in 1969 to give corporate tax status to professional corporations; this in turn has resulted in a significant increase in their number.

[4]Dispensaries were originally independent charitable entities for the treatment of sick poor. They developed in parallel with hospitals and were ultimately displaced by hospital outpatient departments.

persons not requiring hospitalization may receive care; it is usually distinguished from the *emergency room*, although persons with non-urgent problems are often also seen in the latter area, especially during hours when the outpatient unit is not open. It is commonly referred to as the *clinic,* as are its component units, i.e., medical clinic, surgical clinic. (This term is also often used for large group practices, such as the Mayo Clinic.)

Population served is generally a medically indigent one, although middle income levels may be served, especially at university teaching hospitals, and special consultation mechanisms may be available for referring physicians.

Patients are usually seen by house staff (interns and residents) or unpaid attending physicians (voluntary staff).

Increasingly, private patients may be seen by physicians who have offices at the hospital under rental or other arrangements. This is usually distinguished from the general Outpatient Department by a term such as "private ambulatory service."

Health Center. This term has been used to refer to the locus of a wide variety of health care and related activities, and generally implies services to a specific local area, district, or neighborhood. It commonly means a unit of a city or county health department, housing services such as well child and prenatal clinics, and venereal disease and tuberculosis control and treatment units; emphasis is on preventive services.

Neighborhood Health Center. A health center whose purpose is to provide a program of comprehensive health services to a defined local area, often with related social services, and generally with some degree, often considerable, of involvement and participation of members of the local community. The use of non-traditional personnel such as family health workers[5] and emphasis on "health care teams" are characteristic of these centers.

Most were developed in the 1960s with federal funding such as the Economic Opportunity Act,[6] Title V of the Social Security Act (Maternity and Infant Care and Children and Youth Projects), and Model Cities; many are sponsored by local health departments. Some centers are independent but most have some degree of hospital affiliation and may be termed, from the hospital viewpoint, *satellite centers.* A "back-up" hospital is one which provides specialized services and hospital admissions to a neighborhood health center.

---

[5]The family health worker is a new health occupation developed at the Dr. Martin Luther King, Jr. (OEO) Health Center in New York City and described by Harold B. Wise. It is representative of a cadre of newly trained, previously unskilled workers, typically recruited from the communities served. They carry out a variety of delegated nursing, health education, social service and social advocacy functions in health centers and the community. Terminology is diverse and includes community health aides, health guides, neighborhood aides, neighborhood health agents and "out-reach" workers.

[6]Funded the OEO (Office of Economic Opportunity) neighborhood health centers, which were the prototypes of the current neighborhood health center movement.

Analogous programs are the rural health centers developed under federal financing for migrant health and Appalachian development, as well as under OEO and Title V.

Mental Health Center (Community Mental Health Center). A center for the provision of comprehensive mental health services, usually to a defined geographical "catchment" area. It emphasizes the provision of a wide range of mental health services in the community as opposed to the more traditional emphasis of long-term hospitalization of the mentally ill. As defined in federal regulations[7] for purposes of eligibility for funding support, a community health center is one which provides a spectrum of services including, in addition to inpatient services available to the community, outpatient, day care and 24-hour emergency services, and consultation and educational services for community agencies and professional personnel. A community mental health center need not be a physical entity; it can actually be a network of coordinated services. Teams are also emphasized here, as well as short term and "crisis intervention" approaches to treatment. Much use is also made of community workers trained as mental health aides.

"Free Clinics." Neighborhood clinics which provide medical services in relatively informal settings and styles to, generally, students, transient youth, and minority groups. Care is given at no or nominal charge by predominantly volunteer staffs. The first such clinic is considered to be the Haight-Ashbury Free Clinic, organized in San Francisco in the summer of 1967 by David Smith. There are now estimated to be 175-200 such clinics around the country.

Short Stay Surgical Center ("Surgicenter"). An independent,usually proprietary, facility for surgical procedures which do not require overnight hospitalization. The principal rationale for the center is the reduction in costs compared with such hospitalization. The best known is the Surgicenter in Phoenix, established in 1970 by two anesthesiologists, John Ford and Wallace Reid.

Drug Rehabilitation Programs. Programs for rehabilitation of drug abusers are of two major types: *Methadone maintenance*: hospital-related programs for heroin addicts based on the long-term use of methadone as a heroin substitute, supplemented in varying degrees by other rehabilitative services; and *Self-help*: community-based programs, some residential, which emphasize drug-free, group-oriented approaches; the term also often includes a wide spectrum of counseling and "hot-line" services.

---

[7]Under the Community Mental Health Centers Act, 1963.

Visiting Nurse Association (Visiting Nurse Service). A voluntary agency which provides nursing services in the home, including health supervision, education, and counseling; bedside care, and the carrying out of physicians' other personnel such as *home health aides* who are specially trained for specific tasks of personal bedside care.

These agencies had their origin in the visiting or "district" nursing provided to sick poor in their homes by voluntary agencies, such as the New York City Mission, in the 1870s. The first visiting nurse associations were established in Buffalo, Boston and Philadelphia in 1886-87.[8]

"Combined Agency." A nursing agency jointly staffed by nurses from both voluntary (i.e., Visiting Nurse Association) and "official" agencies (i.e., city of county health department).

Home Care Program. An organized program, hospital- or community-based, for the provision of a spectrum of medical services, equipment, and supplies to patients in their homes, generally patients with chronic illness. Community-based programs usually supplement the services of private practitioners; hospital-based programs may provide physician services. The earliest, and still among the best known home care programs, was established in 1947 at Montefiore Hospital in New York City.

X **Home Health Agency.** A term defined in federal legislation (see p. 131) referring to an agency authorized to receive payment under federal programs (Medicare, Medicaid) for services provided in the home. Includes visiting nurse associations and home care programs.

Special Ambulatory Care Personnel

Public Health Nurse (Community Health Nurse). A public health nurse generally works in the community and is concerned with the health of groups and of persons in their usual environment such as home, school, or work. These nurses are most often based in health departments ("official agencies"), schools, or voluntary agencies such as visiting nurse associations. They traditionally function relatively independently and tend to be especially oriented toward the community, the family and the promotion of health and normal development. The nursing staffs of neighborhood health centers typically include public health nurses.

---

[8]See Hanlon, John J., *Principles of Public Health Administration* (References, p. 182) for a good discussion of public health nursing in visiting nurse associations, health departments, and other agencies.

Training includes experience in a community agency, either during a baccalaureate nursing program (as field experience) or after graduation from nursing school. Advanced training formerly obtained by special courses granting a certificate is now obtained via master's degree programs.

Pediatric Nurse Practitioner.[9]   A pediatric nurse practitioner is a registered nurse who has been trained, in a program of four months' (or more) duration, to assume an expanded role in the care of children. This includes comprehensive well child care and the appraisal and management of certain conditions of the acute or chronically ill child. The first formal training program was developed in 1967 by Henry K. Silver and Loretta C. Ford at the Schools of Medicine and Nursing of the University of Colorado. The activities of pediatric nurse practitioners are generally considered to be inherent in present nursing practice in law and ethics and new licensing legislation specific to these practitioners has not been pressed.[10]

Other Practitioners.   More recently, training programs have been developed for "adult (medical) nurse practitioners" and "family nurse practitioners."

"Physician Extenders."   The general concept of "physician extenders" and "assistants for the physician" has attracted wide recent interest in the context of debate, discussion, and program development related to the "health manpower crisis" and the use of "allied health manpower." Terminology, goals, and programs are rapidly changing, and the following few descriptions merely illustrate some of the current trends.

Physician's Assistant (PA).[11]   A physician's assistant is trained to perform a variety of routine and delegated patient services under the supervision or direction of a physician. The first formal training program was established at Duke University in 1966 by Eugene A. Stead. The program comprises nine months' formal instruction and 15 months in clinical rotations, a format which is characteristic of many subsequent programs.

MEDEX.[12]   MEDEX programs are physician assistant programs which were developed specifically for former medical corpsmen with independent duty experience. Their purpose was to train extensions for physicians, especially for general practitioners in rural areas. (Most Medex have been trained to work with specific physicians). The first such program was begun in 1969 by

---

[9] Now often termed *Pediatric Nurse Associate.*

[10] However, in the setting of the general trend toward expanded nursing roles, there has been activity directed toward modification of nursing practice acts to broaden the definition of nursing practice. An example is the 1972 amendment of the New York State statute.

[11] Now sometimes termed *Physician's Associates.*

[12] From the French, "Médecin extension."

Richard A. Smith at the University of Washington, in cooperation with the Washington State Medical Association. The programs generally consist of three months of university training and twelve months of preceptorship.

Child Health Associate. This program was begun in 1969 at the University of Colorado for training child care professionals capable of handling a broad variety of non-life-threatening pediatric problems. This is a five-year program leading to a Bachelor of Science degree. (Two years undergraduate, two years at the medical center, one year of internship.)

Nurse practitioners (see above) are sometimes considered in the physician extender category.

Licensure. The question of legal regulation of assistants to physicians has become an important and controversial one. Many states have recently passed licensing and registration statutes, generally by amending medical practice acts. The earliest were those of California (for physicians' assistants) and Colorado (for child health associates)

Special Terms

"Comprehensive Care". A system which provides a wide variety of health care services, with the implication that these will be coordinated, under the overall direction of a responsible physician or "team" of professionals, and with appropriate attention to preventive and rehabilitative services and socioeconomic factors.

"Primary Care". A term, not yet well-defined, which has gained wide currency since the term *primary physician* was proposed in the report of the Citizens' Commission on Graduate Education in 1966.[13] Its meaning varies from that of "first contact" care (often with the implication of care simple to render, or of evaluation/referral) to that of broad, continuing responsibility for care of individuals or families; it is often used synonymously with family medicine, family practice, or general practice. It is also often used to denote care rendered by internists and pediatricians.

Triage.[14] This term is now commonly being used to describe the sorting out or screening of patients seeking care, to determine which service is initially required, and with what priority. A patient coming to a facility for

---

[13]*The Graduate Education of Physicians,* popularly known as the "Millis Report" after the Commission chairman, John S. Millis. The term was used to denote a physician who would be specially trained to provide comprehensive, continuing, health care. It is now often used as a generic term to refer to general or family practitioners, internists and pediatricians.

[14]From the French, "selecting, sifting," originally applied medically to the sorting of battle casualties.

care may be seen in a "triage," "screening" or "walk-in" clinic. Here it will be determined, possibly by a "triage nurse," whether, for example, the patient has a medical or surgical problem or requires some non-physician service such as social service consultation. Such rapid assessment units may merely refer patients to the most appropriate treatment service, or may also give treatment for minor problems.

Appointment System. The arrangement whereby a patient is given a definite time and date for a visit. *Block appointments* are those given for the same time to all patients, i.e., the beginning of a session; *staggered appointments* are those given for a specific time during a session. These are also referred to as "wave" and "stream" systems. *"Walk-in"* refers to a patient who comes in for care without an appointment.

Screening, Multi-Phasic Screening. Frequently an adjunct of ambulatory care programs; a system whereby a variety of routine tests are performed for the purpose of early disease detection.

Automated Multi-Phasic Health Testing (AMHT). A highly organized system of health testing which includes the use of automated equipment and data processing techniques.

References
Henry K. Silver, Loretta C. Ford and Lewis R. Day, *The Pediatric Nurse Practitioner Program: Expanding the Role of the Nurse to Provide Increased Health Care for Children,* Journal of the American Medical Association, 204:298, 1968.

Eugene A. Stead, *Conserving Costly Talents—Providing Physicians New Assistants,* Journal of the American Medical Association, 198:1108, 1966.

Richard A. Smith, MEDEX, Journal of the American Medical Association, 211:1843, 1970.

Harold B. Wise, E. Fuller Torrey, Adrienne McDade, Gloria Perry and Harriet Bograd, *The Family Health Worker,* American Journal of Public Health, 58:1828, 1968.

Chapter Seven

Voluntary Agencies

Voluntary agencies are private nonprofit organizations whose goals are the amelioration of specific or general health or social welfare problems. They have been developed by private citizen groups, have predominantly lay boards, and usually have professional staff. Many are national bodies with local chapters and affiliates.

Examples of voluntary agencies are the American Cancer Society, American Heart Association, National Tuberculosis and Respiratory Disease Association,[1] and the National Association for Mental Health.

The activities of voluntary agencies are, in general, public education and support of studies, research, and often training in areas of their specific concern. Some also provide direct services (such as the family planning clinics of the Planned Parenthood Federation). Others, usually community based, are organized primarily for direct service; examples of these are family service agencies which provide counseling and other social services, and visiting nurse associations.

The American National Red Cross is unique in being a quasi-official agency, chartered by Congress, and serving as the designated U.S. agency in national and international disaster relief.

There are also a variety of coordinating councils and agencies in which a number of organizations are loosely joined for planning, coordination, mutual education or fund raising purposes. Among these are the local community councils, united funds and community chests, and nationally, the National Health Council.

Also often considered under the rubric of voluntary agencies are the many organizations formed by professionals, agencies and institutions to

---

[1]This is the oldest voluntary health agency, with origins in the Anti-Tuberculosis Society of Philadelphia (1892) and the National Association for the Study and Prevention of Tuberculosis (1904). It was recently renamed the American Lung Association.

further their mutual interests. Examples are the American Medical Association, American Nurses' Association, American Hospital Association, and the Association of American Medical Colleges.

Reference
Robert H. Hamlin, *Voluntary Health and Welfare Agencies in the United States* (New York: Schoolmaster's Press, 1961).

Chapter Eight

Review and Control of Quality and Costs

1. QUALITY CONTROL

A common method of quality control in health as in other fields is the setting of basic minimal standards by public (governmental) and private (voluntary) agencies. The usual mechanisms are those of *licensure* (governmental), *accreditation,* and *certification* (voluntary).

Licensure

The states exercise the extensive licensing powers for health manpower and institutions. By appropriate legislation, the states may authorize persons who meet stated educational and, usually, examination criteria to engage in certain health occupations and professions. In addition to such *mandatory licensure,* some legislation merely authorizes use of a title to those meeting such criteria while not prohibiting others from engaging in the occupation (*voluntary licensure*). About 25 health occupations are licensed in some or all states,[1] either by mandatory (regulation of practice) or voluntary (protection of title) statutes. In addition to setting forth the general criteria, the legislation usually establishes boards of licensure or registration to implement the provisions, make rules and regulations and set procedures. Such boards are made up in large part of members of the profession being licensed.

The stimulus for licensure has traditionally come from professional groups and is often viewed as one manifestation of the process of "professionalization" of health occupations.

---

[1]Examples of personnel under mandatory licensure in all states are physicians, dentists, and pharmacists. Professional nurses have mandatory licensure in most states, but in several only the title (registered nurse) is protected.

193

In addition to such regulation of manpower, the states also license hospitals and other health care institutions. In most cases this authority is vested by the legislature in the state health department. In some instances it is delegated to local city or county authorities.[2]

Accreditation

Accreditation is the process by which an institution or an educational program is determined to meet certain generally accepted standards set forth by an appropriate professional association. It is a voluntary process, and a hospital or program must apply to the accrediting agency for the necessary appraisal.

Examples of such accrediting bodies are the Joint Commission on Accreditation of Hospitals,[3] and the Liaison Committee on Medical Education, a joint committee of the American Medical Association and the Association of American Medical Colleges) which accredits medical schools.

Certification

Certification (or registration)[4] is the process by which individual health personnel are affirmed to have attained a certain level of qualification, according to standards and criteria, such as education, experience and examination, set forth by their professional associations. These may be basic criteria for recognition of individuals as qualified to engage in the occupation, or may be criteria for recognition of advanced qualifications or specialization. An example of the former is the Certified Inhalation Therapy Technician certified by the American Association for Inhalation Therapy; examples of the latter are the medical specialties such as pediatrics and surgery which are certified by the specialty boards affiliated with the American Academy of Pediatrics and the American College of Surgeons.

In addition to these widely prevalent official and quasi-official mechanisms described above, the problem of evaluation and control of the quality of medical programs and institutions has been addressed in many other ways since the publication in 1910 of the most widely known single quality study, the Carnegie Commission's "Flexner Report" on medical education, resulting from a nationwide survey of medical schools.[5]

---

[2] See also pp. 34-39 on the regulation of health institutions.

[3] See p. 25.

[4] The term "registration" may refer, depending on the context, to both licensure and certification. Board of licensure and certification boards are both often termed boards of registration or registries; also, the terms "license" and "certificate of registration" are often used interchangeably.

[5] Indeed, the origins of the Joint Commission on Accreditation of Hospitals lay in the proposals by the Clinical Congress of Surgeons, predecessor of the American College of Surgeons, for an analogous national survey of hospitals.

Medical Audit

Most of these efforts have been variations on the technique of *medical audit* which is broadly defined as the appraisal of quality by medical record review. This commonly has taken the form of analyses of individual cases, with judgments based on defined criteria for diagnosis and management, on expert opinion, or a combination of these.[6]

Professional Activity Study (PAS). The Professional Activity Study was begun in 1953 by the Southwestern Michigan Hospital Council and is now conducted by the Commission on Professional and Hospital Activities.[7] This program pioneered in the application of data processing techniques, first mechanical, then electronic, to the collection and analyses of medical record information on a large scale. Under this program, medical record personnel of participating hospitals abstract standard data from patient records at the time of hospital discharge. The data so obtained is then processed and reported to the hospital in the form of statistical summaries and case by case tabulations. Upwards of 1500 hospitals participate in the Professional Activity Study. The Medical Audit Program (MAP) is a related program whereby data are tabulated by clinical service, and in such a way as to facilitate review of patterns of professional practice.

2. COST CONTROL

Apart from the *claims review* systems long used by health insurance organizations, most of the formal activity related to the control of costs of health services has been by *utilization review*. This has generally been stimulated by concern regarding health insurance costs, and has been largely directed to institutional services, particularly hospital admissions.

Hospital Utilization Committees

It has been a long-time practice, especially during and after World War II, for the medical staffs of some hospitals with shortages of available beds and manpower, to establish committees to monitor admissions, including the setting of priorities. About 1960, however, the number of such committees began to increase, now largely under the pressures of health insurers and others, due to the rising costs of hospital care.[8]

---

[6]This case analysis technique was first exemplified by the "end results" studies of Earnest A. Codman in 1912-1916.

[7]The program has been directed since its inception by Vergil N. Slee under the sponsorship of the American College of Physicians, the American College of Surgeons, the American Hospital Association and the Southwestern Michigan Hospital Council.

[8]The most widely noted early example of such influences was the 1958 order of the Pennsylvania insurance commissioner to three Pennsylvania Blue Cross plans (which

Hospital Utilization Project
of Pennsylvania (HUP)

This is a nonprofit organization sponsored by the Allegheny County Medical Society and the Hospital Council of Western Pennsylvania. It originated in 1963 as a pilot project set up to provide centralized assistance to a number of the area hospital review committees by providing computerized information on hospital discharges. It is an early example of such a regional, computerized process; about 100 Pennsylvania hospitals now use the expanded services of the Project.

Medicare Utilization Review

The Medicare legislation (Social Security Amendments of 1965) required that participating hospitals and extended care facilities have *utilization review plans.* This stipulation lead to the widespread formation of utilization review committees in these institutions as well as to considerable interest in the general problems of such review.

Peer Review

This term is often used for the general process of medical review of utilization and quality, when this is carried out directly or under the supervision of physicians; it often carries the implication that these will be practicing physicians.

Foundations for Medical Care

These are independent corporations sponsored by state or county medical societies which provide one or more services related to third-party payments to participating physicians. Declared common goals are the peer review of costs and quality of care in a fee-for-service context.

All foundations perform some type of review and monitoring of services and fees. Such activities range from review of claims referred by third-party payers (Medicaid programs, Blue Cross, Blue Shield and commercial insurance carriers) to the development of norms for medical procedures, hospitalizations, and length of stay for selected diagnoses. Some foundations sponsor prepaid health insurance plans, principally for employee groups, for which they provide complete claims processing including review and monitoring.

Most of the development of such foundations has taken place since 1965, and much of this since 1970, although the original organization, the San Joaquin Foundation for Medical Care, was established by the San Joaquin Medical Society in 1954. (This is the prototype for the foundations which sponsor complete prepaid health insurance plans.)

---

had requested rate increases) that steps must be taken to control costs. This led to the establishment of utilization committees in many Pennsylvania hospitals.

The *American Association of Foundations for Medical Care* gathers and distributes information about these organizations.

Certified Hospital Admission Program (CHAP)

This program was established in 1969 by the Sacramento California Foundation for Medical Care in cooperation with California-Western States Life Insurance Company. It provides review and certification (for payment) of hospital admissions; the process includes advance review of elective admissions and concurrent monitoring of length of stay.[9] (PAS data for area hospitals was initially used to develop length of stay criteria for the program.) Similar techniques for survey of admissions in advance or early in their course and for monitoring length of stay have become features of a number of other programs.[10]

Professional Standards Review Organizations (PSRO)

The establishment of these organizations was mandated by the Social Security Amendments of 1972 (Medicare-Medicaid amendments). They are associations of physicians organized to review professional and institutional services provided under the Medicare and Medicaid programs. The stated purpose of these organizations is the monitoring and control of both costs and quality.

Among the organizations being designated as Professional Standards Review Organizations are many Foundations for Medical Care.

Experimental Medical Review Organizations (EMCRO)

This term is applied to a number of Foundations for Medical Care and other medical society-sponsored medical review organizations which have been participating, beginning in 1971, in a program sponsored and funded by the National Center for Health Services Research and Development, to develop models for the systematic review of physician services acceptable to professionals, the government and the public.

The EMCRO program was developed in anticipation of the PSRO provisions of the 1972 Social Security Amendments, the language of which mandates the determination of whether the "quality of services meets professionally recognized standards." These are therefore manifestations of a general trend

---

[9]Local (hospital) and regional (area) review committees use varying combinations of *concurrent* review (such as extended duration of stay) and *retrospective* review of hospital and nursing home admissions. The CHAP program adds the additional dimensions of *prior* review and *certification* for payment.

[10]For example, the Hospital Admission and Surveillance Program (HASP) of the Illinois Foundation for Medical Care, established in 1970, which monitors Illinois Medicaid admissions.

toward the integration of techniques for the systematic review of both utilization and quality. (Other examples are QAP[below] and the widespread use of PAS data by utilization review committees.)

Quality Assurance Program (QAP)

This is a program sponsored by the American Hospital Association to expand and strengthen the activities of hospital-based utilization review and medical audit committees.

"Certificate of Need" Statutes

Another recently developed mechanism of cost control is the "certificate of need" legislation which has been enacted by many states. These statutes are directed particularly at control of health facilities construction. Typically, facility construction must be approved by a designated state agency (usually the state health department, often with concurrence of the local [area-wide] comprehensive health planning agency. Evidence that the proposed new or expanded facility is needed by the community must be presented. (See also page 38.)

References

State Licensing of Health Occupations, U.S. Department of Health, Education and Welfare, National Center for Health Statistics, 1967.

Evaluation of the Medical Audit, Paul A. Lembcke, Journal of the American Medical Association, 199:111, 1967.

The Utilization Committee, Vergil N. Slee, in *The Medical Staff in the Modern Hospital,* by C.W. Eisele, Mc-Graw-Hill Book Company, New York, N.Y., 1967.

Foundations for Medical Care, Richard H. Egdahl, New England Journal of Medicine 288:491, 1973.

Chapter Nine

The Pharmaceutical Industry

1. DRUGS

A basic distinction is made between:

1. *prescription drugs* (also *ethical drugs*), which are sold by prescription only and advertising is directed only at the health professionals, primarily physicians; and
2. *non-prescription drugs* (*proprietary drugs, over-the-counter drugs*), which are sold directly to the public without prescription and advertising is directed at the public audience (e.g., aspirin).

The pharmaceutical manufacturers who make and sell prescription drugs refer to themselves as the *ethical drug industry*[1] and the larger firms are represented by the Pharmaceutical Manufacturers Association. The largest U.S. companies include:[2]

Abbott	Pfizer
American Home Products	Richardson-Merrell
Baxter	Schering-Plough
Bristol Meyers	Smith, Kline and French
Johnson & Johnson	Squibb
Eli Lilly	Sterling Drug
Merck & Company	Upjohn
Miles Laboratories	Warner Lambert
Morton-Norwich	

---

[1] Any pharmaceutical is classed as "ethical" if it is advertised only to physicians.
[2] *Fortune,* May 1972; August 1972.

Regulation: The Food and Drug Administration (FDA)

The Pure Food and Drug Act of 1906 specified that certain drugs are to be sold by prescription only and that the federal government is to insure that drug packages accurately state the names and quantities of the active ingredients. Before this time any drug including narcotics could be sold "over the counter" to the public. Impetus for this law came from the American Medical Association and the Muckrakers.

In 1927 the Food, Drug and Insecticide Administration was formed in the Department of Agriculture from the Bureau of Chemistry, which policed drugs prior to this time. In 1938, as a result of 100 deaths from a toxic sulfanilamide preparation, the *Food, Drug and Cosmetic Act* was passed which required that all *new drug applicators* (NDA) be submitted to the government prior to marketing to make sure that adequate toxicity studies had been made (Section 505).

> Required information for an NDA includes a full report on investigations in animals and humans to show that the drug is safe for use, a full statement of the composition of the drug, the method of its manufacture, and samples of labelling.

From 1938 to 1965 more than 14,000 NDAs were received. Special regulations were developed for investigational drugs to be used by experts. This law led to the problem of defining what is a new drug.

In 1953 the FDA became part of HEW.

In 1962, the Kefauver-Harris Drug Amendments were passed as a result of the Kefauver Senate Hearings on drug prices and the Thalidomide tragedy.

This required annual registration and inspection at least every two years of drug manufacturing establishments by the FDA. The FDA is empowered to regulate advertising, and to make a ruling that an NDA is sufficiently *safe* and *effective* before going on the market. The result is that the drug firm must undertake a substantial research and development effort to prepare an NDA.

Biologics

Biologics (biological products, biologicals) are any virus, therapeutic serum, toxin, anti-toxin, or analogous product applicable to the prevention of disease.[3] Biologics, including vaccines and blood plasma products, are regulated by the Bureau of Biologics, a division of the Food and Drug Administration (FDA), which in turn is part of HEW.

---

[3] They differ from drugs in that biologics are usually derived from living microorganisms and cannot be synthesized or readily standardized by chemical or physical means. They tend to be chemically less stable than drugs, their safety cannot be as easily assured and they are never as chemically pure as drugs.

A key regulation in this area is the *Virus-Toxin Law of 1902 (Biologics Control Act)* which was passed as a result of the deaths of a number of children from tetanus, effected by a contaminated diphtheria anti-toxin.

Licenses are granted for the manufacture and sale of biologics and annual inspection by the Division of Biologics Standards is required.

Naming Drugs

Drugs are known by three names:

1. The *chemical name* using the terminology that defines its chemical structure (e.g., 2 methyl-2 propyl-1, 3 propanediol dicarbamate).
2. The *generic name*: The established or official name for the drug (e.g., meprobamate).
3. The *brand name (proprietary drug name)*: The registered trademark of a product given to it by its manufacturer (e.g., Miltown or Equanil).

A drug can be *an entity*: a simple chemical substance or biological product or a *combination.* It can be marketed in different dosage forms (e.g., tablets, syrups, solutions, etc.).

New drugs are patentable. A *patent* is a legal monopoly granted by the federal government for a period of 17 years from the time it is issued. A patent can cover new chemical entities, and new ways of making them, but not drug dosage forms. A company with a patented drug may license other companies to make and sell this drug in exchange for payment (royalties).

The patent is designed as a method for encouraging research and new ideas by allowing the inventor to "capture" the profits from his invention.

2. THE STRUCTURE OF THE PRESCRIPTION INDUSTRY

The central importance of research for new drugs results in large research expenditures. The information and research necessary to process an NDA through the FDA is large and costly. Approval by the FDA and obtaining a patent and a trademark are the start of a marketing campaign which includes advertising to physicians in various forms and visits to doctors by drug detail men, who inform him of the use of this new product.

If there is no patent, other companies may make and sell the drug either under their own brand name or under the generic name. Drugs for sale by generic names are often sold at a substantially lower price. The critics of the industry argue that the difference results in vast monopoly profits from brand name drugs. The defenders of the industry argue that behind the brand name stands the reputation of the company for high quality performance and the price differential reflects quality differences. Usually only large drug firms can undertake this research and marketing process to develop new drugs. Promotional efforts are aimed almost entirely at physicians, who are legally the only ones allowed to write prescriptions.

Outside the hospital, prescriptions are filled only by registered pharmacists working in pharmacies licensed by the state. Pharmacies are either individually or chain owned (e.g., Rexall, Walgreens) and usually run for a profit. They also may provide a wide range of other products for sale which are not related to health. Pharmacists give some advice to patients concerning illness and remedies, particularly in the area of non-prescription preparations.

References

L. Earle Arnow, *Health in a Bottle,* (Philadelphia: J.B. Lippincott Company, 1970). To the extent that anything written on the drug industry is objective and neutral, this is fairly close.

Morton Mintz, *The Therapeutic Nightmare,* (Boston: Houghton Mifflin Company, 1965), 590 pp. A catalogue of horrors. Also, *By Prescription Only,* by the same author.

Prescription Drug Industry Fact Book, Yearly. In praise of the industry.

Reports of the *Task Force on Prescription Drugs,* Office of the Secretary, U.S. Dept. of HEW, especially Final Report, Feb. 7, 1969. Superintendent of Documents, U.S. Government Printing Office.

Appendixes

Appendix A

Alphabet Soup*

A	AAMC	Association of American Medical Colleges/Association of American Medical Clinics
	AB	Aid to the Blind
	ADA	American Dental Association/American Dietetic Association
	AFDC	Aid to Families with Dependent Children
	AHA	American Hospital Association
	ALOS	Average Length of Stay
	AMA	American Medical Association
	AMHT	Automated Multi-Phasic Health Testing
	ANA	American Nurses' Association
	APHA	American Public Health Association
	APTD	Aid to the Permanently and Totally Disabled
	ASCP	American Society of Clinical Pathologists
B	BC	Blue Cross (Sometimes BX)
	BS	Blue Shield
C	CAP	Community Action Program
	CCU	Coronary Care Unit
	CDC	Center for Disease Control
	CHAMPUS	Civilian Health and Medical Program of the Uniformed Services
	CHAP	Certified Hospital Admission Program
	CHP	Comprehensive Health Planning

*This list contains abbreviations noted in the text.

	CONUS	Continental United States (military hospitals)
	C&Y	Children and Youth Project
D	DAT	Dental Aptitude Test
	DDS	Doctor of Dental Surgery
	DMD	Doctor of Dental Medicine
	DO	Doctor of Osteopathy
	DOD	Department of Defense
	DSC	Doctor of Surgical Chiropody
	DVM	Doctor of Veterinary Medicine
E	ECF	Extended Care Facility
	ECFMG	Educational Council for Foreign Medical Graduates
	EDDA	Expanded Duty Dental Assistant
	EEG	Electroencephalograph
	EKG (ECG)	Electrocardiograph
	EMCRO	Experimental Medical Review Organization
	EPA	Environmental Protection Agency
	EPSDT	Early and Periodic Screening, Diagnosis and Treatment
	ER	Emergency Room
	EW	Emergency Ward
F	FDA	Food and Drug Administration
	FLEX	Federation Licensing Examination
	FMC	Foundation for Medical Care
G	GHI	Group Health Insurance Plan
	GP	General Practitioner
H	HASP	Hospital Admission and Surveillance Program
	HEW	Department of Health, Education and Welfare
	HIAA	Health Insurance Association of America
	HIP	Health Insurance Plan of Greater New York
	HMO	Health Maintenance Organization
	HRA	Health Resources Administration
	HR 1	Social Security Amendments of 1972
	HSA	Health Services Administration
	HSMHA	Health Services and Mental Health Administration
	HUD	Department of Housing and Urban Development
	HUP	Hospital Utilization Project of Pennsylvania
I	ICF	Intermediate Care Facility
	ICU	Intensive Care Unit

J	JCAH	Joint Commission on Accreditation of Hospitals
L	LPN	Licensed Practical Nurse
	LVN	Licensed Vocational Nurse
M	MA	Medical Assistance
	MCAT	Medical College Admission Test
	MCH	Maternal and Child Health
	MD	Doctor of Medicine
	MEDLARS	Medical Literature and Analysis Retrieval System
	MIC	Maternal and Infant Care Project
	MPH	Master of Public Health
	MT	Medical Technologist
N	NASW	National Association of Social Workers
	NDA	New Drug Application
	NIH	National Institutes of Health
	NIMH	National Institute of Mental Health
	NLN	National League for Nursing
	NMA	National Medical Association
O	OAA	Old Age Assistance
	OASDI	Old Age, Survivors and Disability Insurance (Social Security)
	OCD	Office of Child Development
	OD	Doctor of Optometry
	OEO	Office of Economic Opportunity
	OMB	Office of Management and Budget
	OPD	Outpatient Department
	OR	Operating Room
	OT	Occupational Therapist
P	PAS	Professional Activity Study
	PGP	Prepaid Group Practice
	PHS	Public Health Service (Also USPHS)
	PMA	Pharmaceutical Manufacturers' Association
	Pod. D.	Doctor of Podiatry
	PPC	Progressive Patient Care
	PSRO	Professional Standards Review Organization
	PT	Physical Therapist
Q	QAP	Quality Assurance Program

R	RMP	Regional Medical Program
	RN	Registered Nurse
	RPh	Registered Pharmacist
	RRL	Registered Record Librarian
S	SNF	Skilled Nursing Facility
	SRS	Social and Rehabilitation Service
	SSA	Social Security Administration
	SSI	Supplemental Security Income
U	UR	Utilization Review
	USPHS	United States Public Health Service
V	VA	Veterans Administration
	VISTA	Volunteers in Service to America
	VNA	Visiting Nurse Association

Appendix B

Chronological List of Laws[1]

1902	Biologics Control Act
1906	Pure Food and Drug Act PL 59-384
1908	Federal Employees Compensation Act PL 60-176
1917	Vocational Education Act PL 64-347
1920	Vocational Rehabilitation Act PL 66-236
1921	Maternity and Infancy Act PL 67-97
1935	*Social Security Act PL 74-271
1943	Vocational Rehabilitation Amendments of 1943 PL 78-113
	Emergency Maternal and Infant Care Act PL 78-156
1944	*Public Health Service Act PL 78-410
1946	*National Mental Health Act PL 79-487
	*Hospital Survey and Construction Act PL 79-725
	*Vocational Education Act of 1946 PL 79-586
1949	*Hospital Survey and Construction Amendments of 1949 PL 81-380
1954	*Medical Facilities Survey and Construction Act of 1954 PL 83-482
	*Dependents Medical Care Act PL 24-569
1958	*Health Research Facilities Act of 1956 PL 84-835
	*Health Amendments Act of 1956 PL 84-911
	*National Health Survey Act PL 84-652
1958	Grants-in-Aid to Schools of Public Health PL85-544
1959	*Federal Employees Health Benefits Act of 1959 PL 86-352
1960	*Social Security Amendments of 1960 PL 86-778
	Graduate Training in Public Health PL 86-720

---

[1] Major laws described or referred to in this book.
*Official short title.

1961	*Community Health Services and Facilities Act of 1961 PL 87-395
1962	Health Services for Agricultural Migratory Workers PL 87-692
1963	*Health Professions Educational Assistance Act of 1963 PL 88-129
	*Maternal and Child Health and Mental Retardation Planning Amendments of 1963 PL 88-156
	*Mental Retardation Facilities and Community Mental Health Centers Construction Act of 1963 PL 88-164
1964	*Hospital and Medical Facilities Amendments of 1964 PL 88-443
	*Economic Opportunity Act of 1964 PL 88-452
	*Graduate Public Health Training Amendments of 1964 PL 88-497
	*Nurse Training Act PL 88-581
1965	*Appalachian Redevelopment Act of 1965 PL 89-4
	*Social Security Amendments of 1965 PL 89-97
	*Mental Retardation Facilities and Community Mental Health Centers Construction Act Amendments of 1965 PL 89-105
	*Heart Disease, Cancer and Stroke Amendments of 1965 PL 89-239
	*Health Professions Educational Assistance Amendments of 1965 PL 89-290
1966	*Comprehensive Health Planning and Public Health Service Amendments of 1966 PL 89-749
	*Allied Health Professions Personnel Training Act of 1966 PL 89-751
1967	*Mental Health Amendments of 1967 PL 90-31
	*Mental Retardation Amendments of 1967 PL 90-170
	*Partnership for Health Amendments PL 90-174
	*Social Security Amendments of 1967 PL 90-248
1968	*Health Manpower Act of 1968 PL 90-490
	Public Health Service Amendments of 1968 PL 90-574
1969	*Federal Coal Mine Health and Safety Act of 1969 PL 91-173
1970	*Community Mental Health Centers Amendments of 1970 PL 91-211
	*Medical Facilities Construction and Modernization Amendments of 1970 PL 91-296
	*Communicable Disease Control Amendments of 1970 PL 91-464
	*Comprehensive Drug Abuse Prevention and Control Act of 1970 PL 91-513
	Public Health Service Amendments PL 91-515
	*Health Training Improvement Act of 1970 PL 91-519
	*Occupational Safety and Health Act of 1970 PL 91-596
	*Family Planning Services and Population Research Act of 1970 PL 91-572
	*Comprehensive Alcohol Abuse and Alcoholism Prevention, Treatment, and Rehabilitation Act of 1970 PL 91-616
	*Emergency Health Personnel Act of 1970 PL 91-623
	*Lead-Based Paint Poisoning Prevention Act PL 91-695
1971	*Nurse Training Act of 1971 PL 92-158
	*Comprehensive Health Manpower Training Act of 1971 PL 92-157

       *National Cancer Act of 1971 PL 92-218
       Social Security Amendments PL 92-223
1972   *National Sickle Cell Anemia Control Act PL 92-294
       *Communicable Disease Control Amendments of 1972 PL 92-449
       *Social Security Amendments of 1972 PL 92-603
       *National Cooley's Anemia Control Act PL 92-714
       *Uniformed Services Health Professions Revitalization Act of 1972
        PL 92-426
       *State and Local Fiscal Assistance Act of 1972 PL 92-512
1973   *Emergency Medical Services Systems Act PL 93-154
       *Health Maintenance Organization Act of 1973 PL 93-222

Index

"A" agency. *See also* 314a agencies, 151, 159, 181
accreditation (educational programs), 54-55, 58, 194
ACTION, 103, 177
administration (health; hospital; health management), 43, 71
  hospitals, 17, 18
  nursing homes, 31
Administration on Aging, 109
admissions, hospital, 11, 23
  emergency, 16
  elective, 16
Advisory Commission on Intergovernmental Relations, 104
Advisory Council on Alcohol Abuse and Alcoholism, 174
Advisory Council on Medical Assistance, 137
Aging, Office of, 108
Agriculture, Department of, 102, 107, 176, 200
aide, 42
Aid To Dependent Children, grants to the states for, 122, 146
Aid to Families with Dependent Children (AFDC), 116, 124, 134, 137, 147
Aid to the Blind, grants to the states for, 123, 124, 134, 146
Aid to the Permanently and Totally Disabled (APTD), 124, 134, 146, 147, 211
Alcohol, Drug Abuse and Mental Health Administration, 109, 111
Alcoholic and Narcotic Addict Rehabilitation Amendments of 1968, 173
alcoholism, 109, 111, 173, 174
allied health personnel, 42, 188-189

Allied Health Professions Personnel Training Act of 1966, 162, 209
ambulance services, 31
ambulatory care, 183-190
  patients, 12
  personnel, 187-189
Ambulatory Medical Care Survey, 113
American Association of Blood Banks, 72
American Association of Foundations for Medical Care, 197
American Association of Homes of the Aging, 25, 30
American Association of Medical Clinics, 184
American Association of Nurse Anesthetists, 70
American Board of Medical Specialties, 59
American Cancer Society, 191
American College of Nurse Midwives, 70
American College of Physicians, 25
American College of Surgeons, 25
American Dental Association, 65
American Dietetic Association, 71
American Hospital Association, 2, 25, 85, 153, 192, 198
American Lung Association, 191
American Medical Association, 25, 34, 58, 75, 183, 192, 194, 200, 212
American Nurses' Association, 70, 192
American Nursing Home Association, 25, 30
American Optometric Association, 73
American Society for Clinical Pathologists (ASCP), 71
  certification of medical technologists, 71-72
ancillary charges; personnel services charges, 12
  personnel, 42

services, 17, 20-21
anesthesiology, 20
Anti-Poverty Program (Economic
    Opportunity Act of 1964), 175-177
Appalachian Laboratory of Occupational
    Respiratory Disease, 113
Appalachian Redevelopment Act (1965),
    103
Appalachian Regional Commission, 103
appointment systems (ambulatory care), 190
areawide comprehensive health planning,
    158, 159
assignment of benefits, 81
    Medicare, 25
    Blue Cross, 173
association (physician practice), 183
Association for Hospital Medical Education,
    113
Association of American Medical Colleges
    (AAMC), 58, 192, 194
Association of University Programs in
    Health Administration (AUPHA),
    71
associations. See voluntary agencies
audiology. See speech pathology
Automated Multi-phasic Health Testing
    (AMHT), 190
auxiliaries (hospital volunteers), 23
available bed days, 12
average daily census. See census
average length of stay, hospital (ALOS), 12

"B" agency. See also 314b agencies, 151,
    159
back-up hospital, 185
bed days. See patient days, hospital
benefits, health insurance, 80, 83
    old age benefits, 122
    Medicare, 126-134, 143, 144
Bennett Amendment, 118
biological products, biologics, 150, 200-201
Biologics, Bureau of, 200
Biologics Control Act. See Virus Toxin
    Law of 1902
Biologics Standards, Division of, 201
biomedical engineering, professions, 43
block grants, 119, 159
Blood Bank, 21
    Blood Bank technologists, 72
Blue Cross, 2, 78, 85-86, 89, 196
Blue Cross Association, 85
Blue Shield, 2, 78, 85-86, 89, 196
Board of health, state, 181
boards (examinations)
    National Boards, 58
    specialty boards, primary, 59
        subsidiary, 61
        conjoint, 61, 63-64

British National Health Service, 77
Budget, Bureau Of. See Management and
    Budget, Office of

Canadian Council on Accreditation of
    Hospitals (CCAH), 25
Capitation (fees), 79
Capitation grants, 119, 164, 165
Categorical grants, 119, 159
census (hospital), 11
Census, Bureau of the, 106
Center for Disease Control, 109, 111
Central Supply (hospital), 19
certificate of need, 38, 179, 181, 198
certification, (manpower). See also
    accreditation, licensure, 42, 59, 61,
    71-76, 194
certification (Medicare), 127, 129, 136
Certified Hospital Admission Program
    (CHAP), 197
certified laboratory assistant (CLA), 72
CHAMPUS (Civilian Health and Medical
    Program of the Uniformed Services),
    102, 109
chaplaincy service, hospital, 22
Child Development, Office of, 108, 109, 177
child health associate, 189
Children and Youth programs (C & Y), 185
    Social Security amendments, 123, 136
Childrens' Bureau, 105, 107, 108, 122
chiropodists. See podiatry
chiropractic services
    professions, 43
    in Medicare and Medicaid, 75, 141
Civil Service Commission, United States,
    103, 174
claim (health insurance), 81
claims (review), 195
    processing, Medicare, 140
clinic (clinic patients), 12, 185
clinical laboratory services, professions, 43
clinical research center, RMP definition,
    156
Clinico-Pathological Conference (CPC), 16
closed panel practice, 79
closed staff, 13
coinsurance, 81, 82
    Medicare, 127, 137, 142, 144
combined agency, 187
commercial insurance companies, 86
Commissioned Corps, United States Public
    Health Service, 106, 148
Commission on Heart Disease, Cancer and
    Stroke, 155
Commission on Hospital Care, 153
Commission on Professional and Hospital
    Activities, 195
committees, medical staff (hospital), 14-15

Communicable Disease Center, 106
Communicable Disease Control Amendments
  1970, 151, 152, 209
  1972, 210
community action programs, 175, 176-177
Community Environmental Management,
  Bureau of, 111, 113
Community Health Service (of HSMHA),
  111
Community Health Services and Facilities
  Act of 1961, 154, 209
Community Health Services, Bureau of, 114
community hospitals, 9
community medicine. *See* ambulatory care
community mental health centers. *See*
  mental health centers, community
Community Mental Health Centers Act.
  See Mental Retardation Facilities
  and Community Mental Health
  Centers Construction Act (1963)
Community Mental Health Centers
  Amendments of 1970, 173, 209
community rating (insurance), 78, 81
Comprehensive Alcohol Abuse and
  Alcoholism Prevention, Treatment and
  Rehabilitation Act of 1970, 174, 209
comprehensive care. *See also* comprehensive
  health services, 189
Comprehensive Health Manpower Training
  Act of 1971, 118, 163, 165, 209
Comprehensive Health Planning Amendments (1967, 1970)
  1967, 160
  1970, 161
Comprehensive Health Planning and Public
  Health Service Amendments of
  1966, 39, 51, 60-62, 85, 151, 158-161,
  209
  sections 314a through 314e, 61-62
comprehensive health planning, state, 159,
  179, 180-181
Comprehensive Health Planning Service, 111,
  114, 161
comprehensive health services, 160, 176
comprehensive health services center. *See*
  neighborhood health centers
comprehensive prepaid group practice, 88
Conference Committees (on legislation), 118
Conference of State and Territorial Health
  Officers, 148
Congressional committees, 119
construction grants, 162, 170, 171-172, 174
consultation (physicians), 16
consumer (definition), 37
Consumer Protection and Environmental
  Health Services, 108
Controlled Substances Act, 174

CONUS hospitals, 516
Cooley's Anemia Programs, 152, 170
cooperative hospitals, 9
coronary care unit (CCU), 19
cost control, 195-198
cost sharing (Medicaid), 139
Council on Medical Education, 59
Credentials Committee (hospital), 15
cultists, 15
customary charges (Medicare), 129

deductible (insurance), 81, 82
  Medicare and Medicaid, 127, 137, 139,
  143-144
Defense, Department of, 102
demand for care, 92
Demonstration Cities and Metropolitan
  Development Act (1966), 102
Dental Aptitude Test (DAT), 65
Dental Auxiliary Utilization (DAU), 66
dentistry (dentists, dental manpower)
  hospital dentistry, 21
  dentists, dental manpower, 44, 65-66
Dependents Medical Care Act of 1956,
  102, 208
detail men, 201
Developmental Disabilities Services and
  Facilities Construction Act, 152
  1970 amendments, 174
dietary services, dieticians, 22
  professions, 44
  dieticians, 71
discharges and deaths (hospital), 11
dispensary, 184
domiciliary institutions, 1, 31, 34, 35
Drug Control Act of 1970 (Comprehensive
  Drug Abuse Prevention and Control
  Act of 1970), 174
drug industry. *See* pharmaceutical industry
drug rehabilitation programs, 102, 186
drugs (prescription, non-prescription;
  chemical, generic and brand names), 21,
  199
  names, 201
dual choice, 37

Early and Periodic Screening, Diagnosis, and
  Treatment (EPSDT) programs, 142
Economic Opportunity Act of 1964, 102,
  175-177, 185, 209
  amendments, 176-177
Economic Opportunity, Office of (OEO),
  102, 175, 176, 185
Education, Division of, 109
Education, Office of, 105, 107, 109, 116
Educational Council for Foreign Medical
  Graduates (ECFMG)
  exam, 60, 62

electrocardiography (EKG, ECG), 22
  technicians, 72
electroencephalography (EEG), 21-22
  technicians, 72
Emergency Health Personnel Act of 1970,
  152, 165, 209
Emergency Maternal and Infant Care Act of
  1943, 208
Emergency Maternity and Infant Care
  Program, 107
emergency medical services, 170
  professions, 49
Emergency Medical Services Systems Act of
  1973, 152, 210
Emergency Service, hospital (emergency
  room [ER], emergency department,
  emergency ward [EW], casualty ward,
  21,185
employee benefit plans, 89, 103
  Social Security, 122
employment taxes (Social Security), 122,
  146
environmental health, professions, 44-45
Environmental Health Sciences, Division of.
  See National Institute of Environmental
  Health Sciences
Environmental Protection Agency, 103, 108
ethical drug industry. See pharmaceutical
  industry
Executive Committee (hospital medical
  staff), 14
Executive Office of the President, 102, 176
exit ("free choice of physician"), 34, 36, 37
Expanded Duty Dental Assistants (EDDAs),
  66
expenditures, national health, 90, 92-100
experience rating (insurance), 81
Experimental Medical Review Organizations
  (EMCRO), 197
extended care facility (ECF), 1, 141
  definition, 3-4
  nursing homes, 29
  Medicare definition, 131
extended care services
  post-hospital, 24
  Medicare definition, 132, 141, 143
externalities (insurance), 78

facilities, health care, 1-39
faith healers, 75-76
family planning services; facilities, 22, 114
  Medicaid, 142, 145
  Public Health Service Act, amendments,
  151-152
Family Planning Services and Population
  Research Act of 1970, 151, 209
Federal Coal Mine Health and Safety Act of
  1969, 209

Federal Employees Compensation Act
  (FECA), 86, 208
Federal Employees Health Benefits Act of
  1959, 103, 208
Federal Employees Health Benefits Programs,
  103
Federal Health Programs Service, 111, 114
Federal Hospital Council, 104, 154
Federal Hospital Insurance Trust Fund, 128
Federal Security Agency, 104, 105, 106,
  107, 146
Federal Supplementary Insurance Trust
  Fund, 129
Federation Licensing Exam (FLEX), 62
Federation of Licensing Boards, 62
fee-for-service, 79
financing, 89-100
  Medicare, 143-144
first dollar coverage, 78, 81
fiscal intermediary, in Medicare, Part A, 128
Flexner Report (1910), 58, 194
Fogarty International Center for the
  Advanced Study of Health Sciences,
  115
folk medicine, 75
Food and Drug Act. See Food, Drug and
  Cosmetic Act (1938)
Food and Drug Administration (FDA),
  105, 107, 108, 109, 113, 200, 201, 202
food and drug protective services, professions, 45
Food, Drug and Cosmetic Act (1938), 107,
  200
Food, Drug and Insecticide Administration,
  200
foreign medical graduates (FMGs), 62
formula grants, 119, 153, 161, 165, 174
formulary, 21
Foster Grandparent Program, 103
Foundations for Medical Care (FMC), 87,
  196, 197
franchising, 38
free clinics, 186
fringe benefits, 89
full-time staff (hospital), 11

genetic blood disorders, 152, 170
grace period (health insurance), 80
Graduate Public Health Training Amendments of 1964, 161, 209
Graduate Training in Public Health Act of
  1960, 161, 208
grand rounds. See rounds
grants-in-aid, 107, 116, 119-120,
  122-123, 148, 150, 151, 158,
  180
Grants-in-aid to Schools of Public Health
  Act, 161, 208

Group Health Association (GHI;
Washington, D.C.), 9, 88
Group Health Cooperative (Puget Sound),
9, 88
group insurance, 81
group practice, comprehensive prepaid,
88, 183-184

Harvard Community Health Plan (Boston),
88
Head Start, 109, 176, 177
Health Affairs, Office of, 102
Health Amendments Act of 1956,
151, 161, 171, 208
health authority, 38
Health Care Facilities Service, 111, 114,
155
health center. *See also* mental health
center, community; neighborhood
health center, 182, 185
health departments, state and local,
181-182
health education and information,
professions, 45
Health, Education and Welfare, Department
of, 101, 104-117, 176, 200
regional offices, 117
Health Examination Survey, 113
health insurance, 80-87
definitions, 78-80
types of policies, 80-81
major forms, 83
characteristics of insured event, 83-85
provision of services, 85
private providers, 85-86
Workmen's Compensation, 86-87
aged and disabled, 115, 123, 126, 139
Health Insurance Benefits Advisory Council,
133, 137, 141, 146
Health Insurance for the Aged. *See also*
Medicare, 115, 123, 126
amended to Health Insurance for the
Aged and Disabled, 139
Health Insurance for the Aged and Disabled
(Social Security Amendments of
1972, Medicare), 139, 146
Health Insurance Plan of Greater New York
(HIP), 86, 88, 184
Health Interview Survey, 113
Health Maintenance Organization (HMO),
36, 78, 79, 87-88, 151, 166, 167,
170
Medicare, 139-140
Health Maintenance Organization Act of
1973, 151, 166-169, 210
Health Maintenance Organization Service,
111
Health Manpower Act of 1968, 163, 209

Health Manpower Education, Bureau of,
109
health plans. *See* Health Maintenance
Organizations; prepaid group practice
health professions and occupations. *See also*
specific occupations, by name, 42-50
education, 56-57
selected descriptions, 71-76
Health Professions Educational Assistance
Act of 1963, 162, 209
Health Professions Educational Assistance
Amendments of 1965, 162, 209
Health Programs Extension Act of 1973,
152
Health Research Facilities Act of 1956,
208
Health Resources Administration, 109,
113-114, 155, 158, 161, 166
Health Resources Development, Bureau
of,
divisions, 114, 166
Health Services Administration, 109, 114,
147
Health Services and Mental Health
Administration (HSMHA), 108, 109, 111
health services development, grants for,
160
HMOs, 166
Health Services for Agricultural Migratory
Workers (1962), 151, 209
health services providers, hospitals, 17
nursing homes, 31
miscellaneous, 49, 50
Health Services Research, Bureau of, 113
Health Training Improvement Act of 1970,
163, 209
Heart Disease, Cancer and Stroke Amend-
ments of 1965, 151, 155-158, 209
Hill-Burton Act. *See* Hospital Survey and
Construction Act of 1946
HMO International (Los Angeles), 88
home care, general; home care programs;
organized home care
hospital-based, 22, 24, 187
home health agency
Medicare definition, 131-132, 187
Home Health Services
Medicare, Part A, 126
Part B, 128
Medicare definition, 132, 140, 143, 144
Public Health Service Amendments, 161,
187
Hospital and Medical Facilities Amendments
of 1964 (Hill-Burton), 155, 209
hospital beds, bassinets (statistics), 11, 32,
34, 35
hospitals, 1
definitions

by type of ownership, 5-9, 33
by type of patient treated, 10
Medicare definition, 130
RMP definition, 156
other, 12-13
general hospital, 2-3, 13-29
departments and services, 17-25
administration, 17-23
flow of work, 25, 26-28
teaching hospital, 11
patient payment status, type of
accommodation, 10-11
hospital statistics, 11-12, 32-33
hospital service charge, 12
Hospital Survey and Construction Act of
1946 (Hill-Burton), 118, 151-155,
180, 208
advisory council on, 104
administration of, 114, 155
summary, 153-154
Hill-Burton amendments, 154-155
Hospital Survey and Construction Amendments of 1949 (Hill-Burton), 154, 208
hospital terminology, 16
Hospital Utilization Project of Pennsylvania
(HUP), 196
house staff; house officers (hospital), 11,
13, 185
Housing and Urban Development,
Department of, 102
H.R.1. See Social Security Amendments
of 1972, 138
Hygienic Laboratory (USPHS), 106

incentive reimbursement, 90
indemnity (health insurance), 81, 86
independent plans (private insurance plans),
86
Index Medicus, 115
Indian Health Service
hospitals, 5, 75, 77, 111, 114
indigent patients, 10
information retrieval systems,
Medicare payment for, 140
inhalation therapy, 22
professions, 49
inpatient care, inpatients, 12, 34
Medicare, 127, 130
(definition), 143
insurance. See health insurance
insurance, hospital (Medicare), 126-128
insurance, supplementary medical (Medicare),
128-130
intensive care unit (ICU), 19, 24
Interior Department of, 103, 107
intermediate care facility (ICF), intermediate care institution, 1, 141
hospitals, 24

nursing homes, 29, 30
Medicaid amendments, 138
Internal Revenue Code, 146
internship, 11, 58-59, 60
Internship Matching Program (National
Intern Matching Program), 59

Job Corps, 175, 176, 177
Joint Commission on Accreditation of
Dental Laboratories, 32
Joint Commission on Accreditation of
Hospitals (JCAH), 25, 34, 130,
133, 140, 194
Joint Commission on Mental Illness and
Health, 171
Joint Conference Committee (medical
staff), 14
Juvenile Delinquency and Youth Develop-
ment, Office of, 108, 109

Kaiser Foundation; Kaiser Foundation
Hospitals, 9, 88, 184
Kaiser-Permanente Plan, 78, 86, 88-89, 184
Kefauver-Harris Drug Amendments (1962),
113, 200
Kerr-Mills Act; Kerr-Mills program. See
Social Security Amendments of 1960

Labor, Department of, 103, 107, 147, 176,
177
laboratories (hospital)
clinical, 20, 31
anatomical, 20
dental, 31-32
professions, 43-44
layman, 37
Lead-Based Paint Poisoning Prevention Act,
209
legislation, health. See also specific legislation by name, 117-119
lepers, 149
Liaison Committee on Graduate Medical
Education, 59
Liaison Committee on Medical Education,
58, 194
library services, professions, 45
licensure, health professions, 42, 189
physicians, 61-62
facilities, institutions, 37-38, 169
biological products, 169
state level, 42, 179, 193-194
long-term care (hospitals). See also extended
care facilities, extended care services,
7, 12

major medical (insurance), 83
Management and Budget, Office of, 102
manpower, health (health personnel), 41-76

career calendar, 56-57
legislation, 161-166, 170
state training programs, 179
Marine Hospital Service, 105,106
Master Facility Inventory Survey, 113
matching grants, 119
Medicaid: 134-135, 145
Maternal and Child Health. *See* Social
Security Amendments of 1965
Maternal and Child Health and Crippled
Children's Services, 125, 135-136,
146
administration, 114
Maternal and Child Health and Mental
Retardation Planning Amendments of
1963 (Social Security Amendments
of 1963), 123, 125-126, 147, 171, 209
Maternal and Child Health Service (in
HSMHA), 108, 111
maternal and child welfare, grants to states
for, 114, 122, 125
Maternity and Infancy Act (1921-1929),
107, 122, 208
Maternity and Infant Care Projects, 125,
185
mathematical sciences, professions, 45
maximum feasible participation, 176
MEDEX, 188-189
Medicaid, 29-30, 116, 121, 123, 126,
134-135, 146, 168, 180, 181, 187,
196, 197
amendments, 124, 137-142
Summary of, 145-146
Medical Assistance (MA),
advisory council, 141
Medical Assistance for the Aged (MAA),
124
Medical Assistance Programs, grants to the
states for (Title 19), 123, 134, 147
medical audit, 194
Medical Audit Program (MAP), 195
medical center (RMP definition), 156
Medical College Admissions Test (MCAT),
58
medical ethics, 35-37
Medical Facilities Construction and
Modernization Amendments of 1970,
155, 209
Medical Facilities Survey and Construction
Act of 1954, 154, 208
Medical Group Management Association,
184
medical library; medical librarian, 22
Medical Literature and Analysis Retrieval
System (MEDLARS), 115
medically indigent (patients), 10, 134, 145,
185
medical records (Medical Records

Department; librarians)
medical staff committee, 15
hospital department, 22
professions, 45, 71
medical schools, 58
Medical Services, Bureau of, 105, 148
medical staff (hospital), 12-15
committees, 14-15
Medical Staff By-Laws, 14
medical technology, professions, 71-72
Medicare, 29-30, 31, 78, 101, 121, 123, 124,
134, 146, 168, 180, 181, 187, 196, 197
Part A (Hospital Insurance Benefits), 89,
126-128, 143
Part B (Supplementary Medical Insurance
Benefits), 128-130, 139 (amended), 144
Part C (Miscellaneous), 130-134
summary, 143-144
amendments, 124, 136-137, 138-142,
(H.R.1)
Medicare Utilization Review, 196
Medicine. *See* physicians, osteopathy
definition, 63
MEDLARS. *See* Medical Literature and
Analysis Retrieval System
Mental Health Act (1946), 171
Mental Health Amendments of 1967, 173,
209
mental health centers, community, 172,
173, 174, 180, 186
Mental Health of Children, 173
Mental Health Study Act (1955), 171
mental retardation, 173
facilities and services, 171-175
legislation, 125-126, 171-175
Mental Retardation Amendments of
1967, 173, 209
Mental Retardation Facilities and
Community Mental Health Centers
Construction Act of 1963, 152, 171-175,
186, 209
summary of titles, 174-175
amendments, 172-174, 209
Mental Retardation Facilities Construction
Act. *See* Mental Retardation Facilities
and Community Mental Health Centers
Construction Act of 1963
methadone maintenance, 186
midwifery, nurse midwife, 46, 47
Migrant Health Act (1962). *See* Health
Services for Migratory Workers (1962)
Mines, Bureau of, 103
model cities programs, 102, 185
moral hazard (health insurance), 84
multiple coverage (insurance), 81

naprapaths, 75
narcotics (addicts, addiction), 150, 173, 175

National Academy of Sciences, 104, 165
National Advisory Cancer Council, 148, 150
National Advisory Council on Health
   Professions Education, 166
National Advisory Council on Nurse
   Training, 166
National Advisory Council on Regional
   Medical Programs, 157, 158
National Advisory Health Council, 148
National Association for Mental Health,
   191
National Association of Clinic Managers.
   See Medical Group Management
   Association
National Board examinations, 58
National Board of Medical Examiners,
   58, 62
National Cancer Act (1937, 1971),
   1937, 106, 150
   1971, 210
National Cancer Institute, 106, 115, 150,
   169
National Center for Family Planning
   Services, 111
National Center for Health Statistics,
   111, 113
National Clearinghouse for Smoking and
   Health, 113
National Communicable Disease Center.
   See Center for Disease Control
National Cooley's Anemia Control Act
   (1972), 152, 209
National Council of Health Care Services,
   30
National Eye Institute, 115, 169
National Federation of Licensed Practical
   Nurses, 70
National Health Manpower Clearinghouse,
   165
National Health Service Corps, 111, 115,
   152, 165, 169
National Health Survey Act of 1958, 208
National Heart and Lung Institute, 115
National Institute of Alcohol Abuse
   and Alcoholism, 111
National Institute of Allergy and Infectious
   Diseases, 115
National Institute of Arthritis and
   Metabolic Diseases. See National
   Institute of Arthritis, Metabolism
   and Digestive Diseases
National Institute of Arthritis, Metabolism
   and Digestive Diseases, 115
National Institute of Child Health and
   Human Development, 115
National Institute of Dental Research, 115
National Institute of Education, 109, 117
National Institute of General Medical
   Sciences, 115

National Institute of Mental Health, 109,
   111, 174
National Institute of Neurological Disease
   and Blindness. See National Institute
   of Neurological Disease and Stroke
National Institute of Neurological Disease
   and Stroke, 115
National Institute of Occupational Safety
   and Health, 111, 113
National Institutes of Health, 104, 105,
   109, 111, 148
   divisions, 115
National Institute on Alcohol Abuse and
   Alcoholism, 111, 174
National Institute on Drug Abuse, 111
National Intern Matching Program. See
   Internship Matching Program
National League for Nursing (NLN),
   68, 70
National Library of Medicine, 115
National Medical Review Committee,
   133, 137
National Mental Health Act of 1946, 208
National Microbiological Institute. See
   National Institute of Allergy and
   Infectious Diseases
National Office of Vital Statistics,
   106
National Research Council, 104
National Research Institutes, 169
National School Lunch Act (1946), 102
National Sickle Cell Anemia Control Act
   (1972), 152, 210
National Tuberculosis and Respiratory
   Disease Association, 191
natural sciences, professions, 46-47
naturopaths, 43, 75
need for care, 92
neighborhood health centers, 115, 176, 177,
   185-186
Neighborhood Youth Corps, 175, 177
New Drug Applicators (NDA), 200, 201
non-cancellable (guaranteed renewable)
   insurance policy, 81
nuclear medicine; nuclear medical technology, 20, 61, 72
   professions, 50
nurse practitioners (including: adult;
   family; pediatric), 188, 189
Nurse Training Act of 1964, 162, 209
Nurse Training Act of 1971, 165-166, 209
nursing, 47, 66-70
   services, hospital, 17, 19
   education, 19, 67-68
   licensure, 68
   specialization, 47, 68-69
   aides, assistants, 69
   public, community health, 187
   legislation for training, 162, 165, 170

nursing care institution. *See also*
    nursing homes; skilled nursing care
    institution, 29-31, 35
    definition, 4
    ownership, 33
nursing homes, 29-31
    licensure of administrators, 31
        ownership, 33

occupancy. *also* occupancy rate, percent
    of occupancy), 12
Occupational Safety and Health Act of
    1970, 103, 209
Occupational Safety and Health Administra-
    tion, 103
occupational medicine, occupational
    therapy, 21, 47, 72
Old Age and Survivors Insurance (OASI),
    107, 123
Old Age Assistance, grants to states for
    (OAA), 122, 124, 125, 134, 135, 146,
    147
Old Age, Survivors and Disability Insurance
    Benefits (OASDI), 115, 123, 126, 138
    (H.R.1), 146
Ombudsman, 37
open staff, 13
optometry (optometrists; opticians;
    ophthalmologists; orthoptists),
    32, 72-73
    professions, 49
orthotic and prosthetic technology,
    professions, 47, 72
osteopathy (physicians; hospitals)
    hospitals, 9
    physicians, 62-63
    other professions, 45-46
outpatient care (institutions; services)
    hospital department, 21, 184-185
    patients, 12
    Medicare payments for, 144
outreach workers, 185

paraprofessional. *See* ancillary personnel;
    professional
partnership (physicians), 183
Partnership for Health. *See* Comprehensive
    Health Planning and Public Health
    Service Amendments of 1966; 1967;
    1970
patient, 201
pathology, 20
patient
    status (by type of payment), 10
    status (by type of accommodation), 10-11
        typical progress through hospital, 26-28
patient days (patient bed days), hospital, 11
payment for care, 77-100
    direct payment, 77

provision of service, 77
insurance, prepayment, 78, 80-87
health plans, 87-89
financing, 89-100
flow of funds, 91
payment of physicians, 79, 128, 140
payment for ancillary services, 20
Peace Corps, 103, 177
pediatric nurse practitioner, 188
peer review, 196
penal institutions, health care in, 149
per diem charge. *See* hospital service
    charge
per diem cost (cost per patient day), 12
Permanente Medical Groups, 88-89
personal care institution, 1
pharmaceutical industry, 199-202
pharmacy; pharmacists
    education, 21, 73
    professions, 47-48
physiatry; physiatrists. *See* physical
    medicine
physical and rehabilitative medicine. *See*
    physical medicine
physical medicine (physiatry; physical and
    rehabilitative medicine; physiatrists,
    physical therapists), 20-21
    professions, 48
    training, 73
    Medicare, Part B, 137, 144
physical therapy. *See* physical medicine.
physician extenders, 188
physicians, 58-65,
    hospitals, 13-14
    education, 58-61
    specialties, specialization, 45-46, 59-61,
    licensure, 61-62
    specialty boards, 63-64
    practice arrangements, 63-64
    Medicare definition of, 132
Physician's Assistant, Physician's
    Associate (PA), 49, 66, 188
Planned Parenthood Federation, 191
podiatry; podiatrists
    professions, 48
    manpower, training, 73-74
Population Affairs, Office of, 151
Population Research and Voluntary Family
    Planning Programs, 151
practical nurses (LPNs), 69
preadmission (prospective screening of
    admissions), 90
preexisting conditions (health insurance),
    80
premium (health insurance), 81, 83
Prepaid Group Practice (PGP), 37, 87-89
prepayment. *See also* payment for case,
    78, 79
primary case, 164

definition, 189
private patients, 10
problem-oriented medical record. *See*
   medical records
professional (*also* paraprofessional; semi-
   professional; sub-professional), 41-42
Professional Activity Study (PAS), 195,
   197, 198
professional corporation (physicians), 184
Professional Standards Review Councils, 141
Professional Standards Review Organization
   (PSRO), 111, 118, 124, 141, 146, 197
Professional Standards Review, Office of,
   111, 147
Progressive Patient Care (PPC), 24
proprietary hospitals, 6, 9, 33
prospective reimbursement, 90
provision of services; provider of services
   (insurance), 85-86, 132, 133
psychiatry; psychiatric services
   Medicare, Medicaid payment for, 142
public health activities, state and local,
   179-182
   state public health departments, 180-181
public health, careers in, 74, 161-166
Public Health Service, United States
   (USPHS), 59, 105-107, 108, 109-111
   122, 147, 153, 169, 177
   hospitals, 57
   health manpower development, 114
   administration, 148
Public Health Service Act of 1944, 106,
   147-152, 159, 166, 208
   amendments, 151-152, 157 (1968; 1970)
   summary of titles, 169-170
Pure Food and Drug Act of 1906, 200, 208
Pure Food, Drug and Cosmetics Act, 113

quacks, 75
quality assurance, in Public Health
   Service Act, 168, 169
Quality Assurance, Bureau of, 115
Quality Assurance Program (QAP), 198
quarantine, 111, 113, 150
queue, 85

radiology (*also* radiologists, radiologic
   technicians), 20
   professions, 58
   manpower, training, 74
realized demand (for care), 92
reasonable charges (Medicare, Part B),
   128
   amendments, 137
reasonable cost
   in Medicare, Part A, 127
   Part B, 129
   Medicaid, 135
   Maternal and Child Health, 136

Red Cross (American National Red
   Cross), 104, 191
referral, 16, 38
regionalization, regional planning, 38-39
Regional Medical Programs (RMP), 114,
   151, 155-158
   definition, 155
   amendments, 157-158
Regional Medical Programs Service, 111,
   114, 158
registered nurses (RNs), 67
regulation (health services institutions). *See*
   also licensure, 34-39, 179
   types of, 36
rehabilitation services, professions, 48
reimbursement formula, 90
reinsurance, 84
relative value scale (fees), 79
renal dialysis (kidney dialysis), 22
renal disease, chronic, *under* Social
   Security, 142
Research and Statistics, Office of, 116
research grants, 119
residential facility, 29-30
residency training, 58-59, 60
Retired Senior Volunteer Program, 103
retrospective denial of payment, 90
revenue sharing, 119
rider (insurance), 80
rounds (ward rounds, teaching rounds,
   grand rounds), 16
Ross-Loos Medical Group (Los Angeles),
   88

Saint Elizabeths Hospital, 105-151
San Joaquin Foundation for Medical Care,
   196
satellite centers, 185
scholarships and loans. *See* training grants
screening
   multi-phasic, 142, 190
   child health (Medicaid), 145
secretarial and office services, medical,
   professions, 48
self-care patients (hospital), 24
self-help (drug rehabilitation), 186
self-pay patients, 10
semi-private patients, accommodations,
   10, 11
   under Medicare, 132
semi-professional. *See* professional
service benefits, 86
short-term care (hospitals), 8, 12

Shriners hospitals, 6, 9
Sickle Cell Anemia Program, 152, 170
skilled care services; facilities, *in*
  Medicare, Medicaid, 140, 143
skilled nursing care; facilities (SNF), 29-30
  in Medicare, 127, 131, 140, 141, 143
sliding fee scale, 79
slip law, 118
Small Business Administration, 176
Social and Rehabilitation Service, 108, 109,
  147
  divisions, 116
  Medicaid, 145
social sciences, professions, 48
Social Security Act of 1935, 29, 106, 107,
  121-123, 208
  original titles, 122
  summary of titles, 146-147
  administration, 147
Social Security Administration, 105, 107,
  109, 115-116, 146, 147
  divisions, 116
Social Security Amendments *of* 1939,
  1950, 1956, 123
  1960 (Kerr-Mills Act), 123, 124-125, 134,
  208
  1965 (Medicare, Medicaid, Maternal and
  Child Health), 126-136, 195, 209
  1967 (Medicare, Medicaid amendments),
  136-142, 209
  1971, 138, 210
  1972 (H.R. 1), 29, 118, 138-142, 197, 210
Social Security Board, 107, 121, 122, 146
Social Services (*also* social work, social
  workers)
  hospital, 22
  professions, 48
  manpower, training, 74-75, 141, 181
solo practice, 183
Special Action Office for Drug Abuse
  Prevention, 102
specialized rehabilitation services,
  professions, 48
specialties, specialization. *See* physicians
speech pathology (audiology), 22
  Medicare 141, 144
  professions, 48
spell of illness (Medicare definition), 130
staffing ratio (hospitals), 12
State and Local Fiscal Assistance Act
  of 1972, 120, 210
State Services, Bureau of, 105, 148
statistics, hospital, 11-12
subprofessional. *See* professional
subsidiary boards (subspecialization), 61
super agencies. *See* umbrella agencies
Supplemental Security Income for the
  Aged, Blind and Disabled, 115, 124,
  142, 146, 147

support services, hospital, 17, 23-24
Surgeon General, Office of, 148
surgical center, short stay (surgicenter), 186
survey reports, 142

target population, hospital, 10
technician assistant, 42
technologist, 42
therapist, 42
third party payers
  patient status, 10
  financing, 90
314a agencies ("A" agencies), 39, 159, 164
314b agencies ("B" agencies), 39, 158,
  159, 164
time limits (insurance), 80
Tissue Committee (hospital), 15
Title 5. *See* Maternal and Child Welfare,
  grants to states for
Title 18. *See* Medicare
Title 19. *See* Medicaid
TPR (temperature, pulse, and respiration),
  15
training grants, 119, 158, 160, 161-166
  170, 172, 173
Training in Expanded Auxiliary Management
  (TEAM), 66
triage, 189

umbrella agencies, 182
unemployment compensation (insurance),
  107
  Social Security, 122, 146, 147
Uniformed Services Health Professions
  Revitalization Act of 1972, 210
unit manager, 19
upper limit on coverage (insurance), 80, 82,
  83
usual and customary fee, 79
utility regulation, 38
utilization review, 14, 130, 132, 140, 143,
  196
  hospital medical staff committee, 195,
  Medicare definition, 131

vendor payments, 90, 123
Veteran's Administration, 5, 104
  hospitals, 6-7
veterinary medicine, professions, 49, 75
Virus-Toxin Law of 1902, 201, 208
Visiting Nurse Association (VNA), Visiting
  Nurse Service, 187
VISTA. *See* Volunteers in Service to
  America
Vital Statistics, Division of, 106
Vocational Education Act of 1917,
  208
Vocational Education Act of 1946,
  161, 208

Vocational Rehabilitation Act, 69, 200
    amendments (1943), 108, 208
Vocational Rehabilitation, Office of
    105, 108
vocational rehabilitation programs, 107,
    122, 180
    professions, 49
voice (regulation), 34, 36, 37
voluntary agencies, hospitals, 6, 8-9,
    33, 191-192
voluntary staff, 185
Volunteers in Service to America (VISTA),
    103, 175, 176, 177

waiting list (hospital), 12
waiver (insurance), 80
ward clerk, 19
ward patients, 10, 11
Weed Lawrence L., M.D., 16
Welfare Administration, 108
work training and work study programs
    (Economic Opportunity Act),
    175, 176
Workmen's Compensation, 86-87

X-ray. See radiology

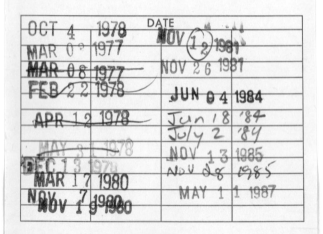

	DATE	
OCT 4 1978	NOV 1 2 1981	
MAR 0 1977		
MAR 08 1977	NOV 2 6 1981	
FEB 2 2 1978	JUN 0 4 1984	
APR 1 2 1978	Jun 18 '84	
	July 2 '84	
MAY 3 1978	NOV 1 3 1985	
DEC 1 3 1978	NOV 28 1985	
MAR 1 7 1980	MAY 1 1 1987	
NOV 7 1980		
NOV 1 9 1980		

003085

© THE BAKER & TAYLOR CO.